I0146193

MENTAL HEALTH FOR
MILLENNIALS
Vol 5

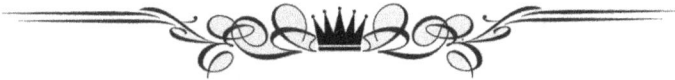

'On Resiliency'

Founding and Series Editors
Dr. Niall MacGiolla Bhuí
Dr. Phil Noone

BOOKHUB

PUBLISHING

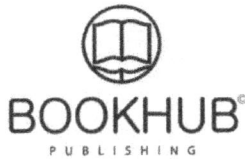

Published by Book Hub Publishing, An Independent Publishing House with
Offices in Galway and Limerick, Ireland.
Book 5 in the DissertationDoctorsClinic 'Millennials' Series

www.bookhubpublishing.com
www.dissertationdoctorsclinic.com
www.thedoccheck.com
@BookHubPublish @ThesisClinic

Copyright Individual Authors & Book Hub Publishing (2021).
Each Author asserts the moral right to be identified as the author of their work.
Dr. Niall MacGiolla Bhuí and Dr. Phil Noone are Series Editors (2017-2023).
Giselle Marrinan, M.Sc. is co-Editor on this collection of Essays. She has also
ghost-written two chapters with contributors.
ISBN: 978-1-7399578-4-1

Sectional Break Photography by Niall MacGiolla Bhuí

About the Clinic Series

The purpose of this DocCheck.Com Mental Health For Millennials Series is to encourage us all to read current material on various themes related to millennial life that is grounded in experience, with a backdrop in theory, written in a style that is fully accessible, interesting and genuinely meaningful to the daily experiences of us all. This is book five of our series with two more books scheduled to follow (2017-2023). We included the guest chapters in this book because we all believe the theme of resilience, in the context of millennials, deserves greater attention.

With the global pandemic of COVID-19, we have all been forced to look into ourselves, to draw from our resiliency (the theme of this book) and to reimagine how and why we engage as we do with the world and our communities. This is as true for millennials as for any other demographic.

Our aspiration is that these books will facilitate readers to understand in a little more detail, the dynamics of millennial life as it is experienced, through providing frameworks for conceptualization and practice.

This series is designed to be useful for: 1) the individual looking to enhance his/her knowledge about millennials and mental health and wellness 2) the interested professional who does not want to read purely theoretical material.

And, make no mistake; lives are complex for millennials. The age of the Internet and 'wearable technologies' presents many challenges - some foreseen but, oh so many, not so. In all of this, millennials are trying to make sense of themselves and their lives and we are trying to make sense of them (that's the older contributors in this book. We've also included some millennials for balance).

Every generation brings with it specific challenges and some people are more adept at change than others. The series itself is intended, therefore, not just to be 'books to read' but also as reference guides for practitioners, family support workers and mental health teams. Feel free to dip in and out of whatever chapter takes your fancy. We're not precious about individual chapter ownership and include essays on a range of topics. Happy reading.

Dr. Niall MacGiolla Bhuí

Table of Contents

CHILDREN, YOUTH AND RESILIENCE

FROM THE ARCHIVES

CREATIVE WRITING

'On Resiliency'
The Open Water

> We meet no
> **ORDINARY PEOPLE**
> *in our lives.*
>
> *C.S. Lewis*

Escaping from a Diagnosis of Disconnection: Our Pod of Three Take to the Sea Embracing the Wild Atlantic Way & Resiliency

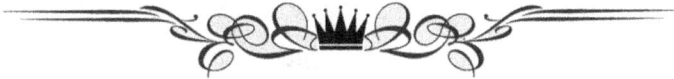

Dr. Niall MacGiolla Bhuí

No talk is ever given without first indicating your humility. "I am an ignorant man; I am a poor man" – all the talks start this way – "I don't know nearly as much as you men sitting around here, but I would like to offer my humble opinion", and then he'll knock you down with logic and wisdom.

— Allen C. Quetone, Kiowa

Introducing Resilience

Back in the day I researched a doctorate on the theme of resilience in psychology. Over a three year period, it took me to special projects, youth offender centres and prisons from Limerick to Cork to Tipperary to Dublin. It also took me to a beach in Kerry, Ireland with a cohort of research participants from inner city Limerick and I've never forgotten their pure joy at being out in nature, running and

1

stumbling in equal measure over sand dunes and then, in the afternoons, swimming in the cold, cold, cold Atlantic Ocean when their usual landscape was one of concrete and steel.

UK domiciled, Dingle man, Alan Creedon (2021) has a beautiful passage in his book where he states of his home place in Kerry, "It is a stunning place and a tough place in many ways. It's fantastic for storms, watching those big rollers coming in can be an awesome sight and sound. It's a place of raw, unspoilt nature, which gets into a person, there's no doubt. It's possible to feel separate from the rest of the world there. Seabirds are plentiful, grass capped sandstone cliffs and brown-gold sandy beaches define the boundary between land and sea. And on a warm summer day it's the most beautiful place in the world when you see the sun sparkle on the gently rippling ocean." Such a landscape speaks of many locations around the south, west and north west of Ireland. These are our places of refuge in this time of pandemic.

A Time of Disrupted Belonging

One of the most prominent psychiatrists of recent times, Dr. Karl Menninger, contended that modern youth suffer from what he termed 'disrupted belonging'. He noted that in earlier times, children and youth were nurtured by extended family, church, and community but that today, many detached young people seek 'artificial belongings'. The resulting epidemic of emotional disorders is described by psychiatrist Edward Hallowell (1999) as the 'diagnosis of disconnection' (cited in Brendtro and Long, 2005: 66).

A sense of disconnection is now all around us with COVID-19 seeping into practically every social interaction be it study groups, work groups, whilst having dinner, in shops, businesses and on every mode of public transport. But, there's one place I've found to be disconnection free – the ocean. Here I can embrace resilience.

Ann Masten defines resilience as a 'class of phenomena characterised by good outcomes in spite of serious threats to adaptation or development' (2001: 228) and it is commonly considered that there are two types of resilience, unhealthy and healthy. 'Healthy' resilience is expressed through pro-social, compassionate, harmonious, adaptive behaviours. In contrast, 'unhealthy' resilience is seen in the use of aggressive, controlling, withdrawing, or self-destructive behaviours (Brendtro and Long, 2005).

I actively chose in January 2021 to, once again in my life, embrace healthy resilience when I got an offer via message (how else?) from millennial friend, Cliona, to come join her and another great friend of mine, Phil, for an ocean swim. 'What the hell?' I thought to myself, 'It's January and it's freezing outside'. I then reflected on the invitation and somewhat hesitantly replied…'Would love to'. I didn't realise it then, but that text fundamentally changed how I was coping with COVID-19 and my mental health. Eight months later, our swimpod3 is still busy swimming off Blackrock Diving Tower. More of that later in the chapter.

Resilience is a term really used to describe a set of qualities that foster a process of successful adaptation and transformation *despite* risk and adversity (Benard, 1991). Persons who are resilient have the capacity to withstand, overcome, or recover from serious threat (Masten, 2001). Simply put, resilience is the ability to bounce back from adversity. Resilience is not simply an *absence* of psychological symptoms despite having experienced adversity, it is the possession of a positive adaptive ability that enables a person to feel competent despite risky living conditions (Sagy & Dotan, 2001).

The open sea is certainly a risky environment and it is in that space I have come alive again over the government imposed pandemic response lockdown of 2021. But, for me to understand why I have returned to the sea this year, it's important to go back to my childhood. Oh, my psychotherapist friends must be rubbing their hands in glee.

Confronting 'Disrupted Belonging': The Slanted, Sideways Rain of Galway

I've swum all my life; rivers, lakes, ponds, pools and the sea. It didn't and still doesn't matter. I carry a wet bag in the boot of my car with goggles, a towel, shorts and a wetsuit from my Triathlon and Ironman days. If there's water and it's deep enough, well then, it's worth exploring and there are so, so many beaches along the west coast of Ireland. I've always loved the feeling of gliding under water, the sensation of the cold, the sights of the sand or stones shimmering under me. It's hard to believe now, but as kids in St. Pats Primary School in Galway City, in the Spring and Summer evenings we swam for hours in the filthy canal that broke the journey from our home in St. Mary's Road to the school in town.

We delighted in jumping in off the bridges that dotted the way from Claddagh up to what is now NUIG. We sometimes mitched school on particularly warm days and, a couple of times, one of our favourite teachers at the time might join us muttering, "Say nothing lads." Good times. Of course, we said nothing.

Speaking of resiliency, I don't ever remember any of my three brothers or friends ever falling ill with infections from our canal escapades in the murky and reedy waters. We were more terrified of potentially getting bitten by eels (and you can guess where we were most afraid of being bitten as pre and barely teens) and mindful of those dangerous reeds. When bored of the canal water, we would seek out open sea water and would often walk or cycle up to Blackrock in Salthill and spend an entire day, regardless of the weather, hopping off the Tower daring each other into contortionist acts of bravery - or was it stupidity? Happy times.

COVID-19, Disconnection and Connection(s)

Here's an interesting fact. The average air temperature in Galway in January and February is between 3 degrees and nine degrees. The average sea temperature is just 9.6 degrees so why, oh why, would anyone desire to wade through the sideways, slanted rain and wind of our little coastal community, strip off, and start swimming in the froth bowl that is Blackrock in Salthill? One answer is, it's a challenge. A challenge of one's resolve, determination and staying power. It's also backed by science and my friend, colleague and seaswimpod member Dr. Phil Noone mentions the work of Wim Hof in her chapter. Perhaps it is more about friendships and trust with one's swim partners. Connections and connecting at a time of profound disconnect, of sustained hate and haters across all the virtual platforms with a new international and national pastime of calling each other out and cancelling diverse opinion.

At the time of writing this chapter, COVID-19 is devastating economies and the social and personal fabric of societies the world over. We are no different in Ireland. We await the various vaccines, some with open hands and others rather begrudgingly. We are daily inundated on the news, in newspapers, on TV, on radio and on social media with advice as to what we should take, what we can do, what we should not do to 'avoid the virus'.

So, what to do? We pod of three long-term friends, Phil, Cliona and I, decided to sea swim our way through January 2021 as an exercise in wellness and resilience. And that's just what we did…So, two oldies and one millennial. What could possibly go wrong?

Physiology of Open Water Swimming

There is no doubt that exercise increases our happiness. Physiologically, there is an immediate increase in our heart rates when we exercise. Our brains recognise this change as stress and respond to it. A protein called Brain-Derived Neurotrophic Factor (BDNF), is released which helps protect and repair our memory neurons. We release endorphins which block the discomfort of exercise and make us feel, well, euphoric. Who needs the dance floor when you have the cold, cold water of the Atlantic? My own view of happiness is more about a sense of calm than the chase for and obtaining material things.

There is now a very established body of science that has examined the benefits of open sea swimming (Hof, 2020). It's not a good idea to swim open water by oneself (I got a really bad cramp in my left thigh when competing in an Olympic Triathlon one year and had to drag myself through the water to make it to the safety of a pier) so there is a great sense of comradery when swimming with a group of friends. We are social beings. We need to interact in the real world with real people. It is here we find deep connections in the deep water.

The Ocean Calls our Names

Day after day, the three of us in our little protected seaswimpod braved wind, rain, hail and eventually amazing sunshine to get into the open water. There were days when none of us wanted to swim, when we wanted to stay in our respective homes on our respective couches with coffee in hand and a good book for company. But, we would text each other and issue the usual invitation 'Swimming this afternoon guys' and we would get up, get dressed and show up. We would walk our 7k first and then strip off and merge into the water. It was, and remains, a feeling of accomplishment to complete what on the surface appears to be such a mundane thing, but you know what? It has become a truly joyful, transformative experience. We are now swimming a kilometre+ each time, we have, quite literally, left the safety of the shore and embraced uncertainty in these COVID-19 times.

We notice there are more and more millennials swimming since the weather has improved. Many of them have also found calm in the sea, comradery in their swim groups and a rest from the constant negativity. Try it. You won't be disappointed. And, gratitude to Cliona for her text last January. Turns out millennials have excellent ideas. And are resilient.

References

Brendtro, L and Long, N. (2005). Reclaiming Children and Youth. Vol 14, Issue 2 (Summer 2005): 66-68.

Creedon, A. (2021). *The Search For Still Waters*. Galway: Book Hub Publishing.

Benard, B. (1991, August). Fostering Resiliency in Kids: Protective Factors in the Family, School, and Community. Portland, OR: Northwest Regional Educational Laboratory.

Hallowell, E. (1999) Cited in Brendtro, L and Long, N. (2005). Reclaiming Children and Youth. Vol 14, Issue 2 (Summer 2005): 66-68.

Hof W. (2020) The Wim Hof Method. Activate Your Potential, Transcend Your Limits. London: Ebury Publishing.

Masten AS. (2001). Ordinary magic. Resilience processes in development. Am Psychol. 2001 Mar;56(3):227-38. doi: 10.1037//0003-066x.56.3.227. PMID: 11315249.

Sagy S, Dotan N. (2001). Coping resources of maltreated children in the family: a salutogenic approach. Child Abuse Negl. 2001 Nov;25(11):1463-80. doi: 10.1016/s0145-2134(01)00285-x. PMID: 11766011.

'Blue-Space' Connectedness and Building Resilience

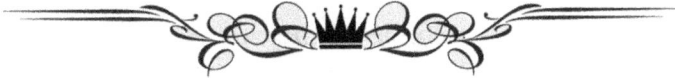

Dr. Phil Noone

"The voice of the sea,
a Soul keeper,
a Soul speaker,
always"

(Noone 2021).

Introduction

'Blue-space' is a very beautiful term often used to describe how we experience time spent in or at oceans, rivers or other water-landscapes. Even saying the word 'blue-space' draws me into the wonders and imaginings of spending time in water. I have always been an avid swimmer and water sports enthusiast, spending much time surfing, scuba diving, kayaking and swimming in the Australian and Irish oceans. For me, blue spaces offer solitude and connectedness that act as positive resilience enhancers. So, what of Millennials? How is it for them? Included here is my own personal experience peppered with insights from psychological and sociological research.

Dr. Phil Noone

Personal Experience January 2021

I need to get away, to be alone. Solitude! My head is bombarded with news, media reports of Covid 19: Cases rising. Lives Lost. Ireland in Level 5 restrictions. Third nationwide lockdown to continue. Job losses to increase. Anxiety and depression levels increasing amongst Millennials...

Realising my need to escape the whirling noise in my head of uncertainly, chaos, negative news feeds, what sociologist Bauman calls our liquid, everchanging, fragmented world (Bauman 2002) and Beck as 'risk society' (2005). And how right they are, neither of them writing about our current pandemic crisis!!

I rise early. I shiver. It's cold. A frosty, minus 3 degrees. I wrap up warm. Boots, hat, gloves. Ready. I drive to the Claddagh in Galway. Park my car. Emerge into the dark, Angel, the dog for company. My breath frosted and white. It takes a minute to settle. To adapt to the cold. But, oh, the magic of it. The stillness. Alone. I walk. Hearing the seagulls as they circle above me. The pant of the dog as she runs alongside me.

It's getting light. I hear some joggers in the distance. Chatting. They pass. We greet. Move on. I hear the sea. Lapping against the rocks. Slowly, silently, the day opens, like a dungeon door, its hinges oiled. Transient darkness. And then the slow beginnings of sunrise. I walk along. Reach the beach. Stretch of white sand. I sit. Needing to be still. This moment too magical to move. I lie. Prop my head on my rucksack. And silently watch the sunrise. In this cold wintery morning.

Cognitive thoughts come and go. Christmas, company, festivities, snippets of conversation. Embracing it all, I let it go. Thoughts of lockdowns, zooms, remote working come and go. In this 'solitude-space' I am me. I am still. The air is still. The energetic activity of the day not yet begun. My mind settles. And I tune into the visceral experience of now. My awareness of the sun rising magnifies. Colours gradually changing-

10

white, orange, red. I move. Rest against a rock. Too beautiful to get up and walk. Motionless. I remain. Silent. Appreciating this solitude, allowing it to soak into my inner being. Capturing resilience, holding it, embracing it, allowing it to settle. Allowing me to settle. Once again whole, strong, ready for the new day.

This experience made me curious about solitude, what it is, how it is conceptualised, its benefits and how millennials use solitude in their cultural world. It also led me to marvel at the power of the 'blue-space', either swimming in the sea or just resting silently by the 'ocean-blue'.

What is Solitude?

Solitude is defined as a psychological experience of being alone (Larson, 1990), expanded by Nguyen et al. (2017) to include, without communication, stimuli, and activities or devices that might facilitate virtual communication such as text messages or social media.

Although relatively new to modern culture, solitude in nature is an ancient form of ritual and ceremony used in indigenous cultures worldwide (Noar & Mayseless, 2020) Nineteenth-century anthropologists and cultural historians used the term 'vision quest' to describe ceremonial practices where individuals spent prolonged periods of time alone to find their individual strengths and purpose in life (Gennep, 1960). But the notion of solitude has also been stigmatised, viewed as an inconvenience, a punishment, something to avoid or the domain of loners (Crane, 2017). In more recent times, solitude is viewed as having psychological and therapeutic benefits especially when pursued by choice and is a powerful tool that can enhance the strengths and capacities inherent in a cohesive self (Noer & Mayseless, 2020). Furthermore, they suggest that solitude can act as an antidote to the loneliness, stress and depression on the rise in our modern culture, often linked to our over stimulated urban environments and lifestyles. Overall, there is much empirical and theoretical literature that points to solitude as a means for profound personal growth, to new ways of knowing oneself, to enhancing our sense of connectedness and ultimately our sense of personal belonging and purpose.

What Occurs when we are Alone?

Merton, a Trappist monk and writer who spent long periods of time alone, believed that:

"We cannot see things in perspective until we cease to hug them to our bosom" (Merton 1958).

Coplan et al. (2014) suggest that being alone provides a gateway to a deep internal process that offers us the space to explore our relationship with ourselves. And this, in turn, alters our relationship with others and the world we live in. I believe it acts as a connectedness conduit. It enhances our sense of the BPC model of connectedness (Be-Present-Connect) (Noone, 2019). But to be present, we need to be still, to be silent, to allow for self-discovery, to allow for the cognitive freedom away from the daily demands of human experience. For me, solitude and Mindfulness Meditative Practice have a similar impact, but I acknowledge, this is very much my individual experience and interpretation.

So what about Millennials?

Millennials are a group born between 1980 and 1996, expected to have reached adulthood by the turn of the 21st century. In Japan, the term 'nagara-zoku' is used for Millennials, translated as 'the people who are always doing two things at once'. Millennials are considered digital natives, always connected to social media and the digital world. Delmar, writing in

The Irish Times (2018), describes Millennials as the overstimulated generation and argues that excessive screen use boosts the release of stress hormones and increases nervous system arousal. Sleep becomes disturbed which, in turn, can result in increased agitation. Switching 'off' is happening less as young people remain permanently 'on', living in an adrenaline fuelled way.

The recent Deloitte Global Millennial and Generation Z Survey Report (www.Deloitte.com/millennialssurvey 2021), conducted with 1465 Millennials in 45 countries across North America, Latin America, Western Europe, Eastern Europe, the Middle East, Africa and the Asia Pacific showed that pre-pandemic 44% of Millennials felt stressed all or most of the time. Yet, a follow up report indicated that stress levels had dropped 8% points for Millennials during the early phase of the pandemic. This may have occurred due to changes in lifestyle, such as reduced commute to work and a simpler lifestyle. But as the pandemic persisted, the sense of relief that may have been felt at the start, lessoned and a return to pre-pandemic stress levels occurred, with 44% of Millennials reporting feeling stressed all the time. Their main concerns focused on their uncertain financial futures, job and career prospects in addition to family well-being. These concerns were more prevalent in women who experienced greater job losses and increased family caring responsibilities during this time. In terms of coping with the pandemic, though frustrated and impatient with the restrictions, undercurrents of optimism persisted.

Recent research conducted by Nguyen et al. (2017) published in the Society for Personality and Social Psychology reported that solitude can lead to relaxation, reduce the impact of stress, especially when people choose to be alone. With a sample of 173 undergraduate students aged 18-22 years, using diaries and surveys as data collection methods, showed that solitude can be used to regulate affective states such as calmness and anger.

Interestingly, having choice or feeling autonomous is an important meditator in whether the psychological impact of solitude is positive or negative. This study also showed that if participants practiced solitude for 15 minutes per day for as little as a week, the perceived benefits had some spill over to the following week.

Resilience and the Power of 'Ocean-Blue'

Resilience is our capacity to bounce back from or cope with adverse events in life (Barry, 2018). During the Covid pandemic, restrictions lead to a reduction in our social space, cultural outlets were closed, remote working with its challenges continued, and for many, a sense of isolation and loneliness potentially swamped us. As indoor swimming pools were closed, SwimPod3 was formed and we decided to take the plunge and jump in!! Into the cold Atlantic waters at Blackrock diving tower in Galway, on the Wild Atlantic Way, West Coast of Ireland.

Research has shown that spending time in blue spaces provides numerous health benefits, to include mental health and psychosocial well-being (Kelly 2021; Hof 2017; 2020; Carney 2017) Evidence from a systematic review conducted by Britton et al (2020) showed that blue spaces had positive benefits for social connectedness, in particular a sense of belonging and interaction with others who have shared life experience. The amazing Eskey Britton, a marine social scientists at NUIGalway, an internationally renowned big wave surfer and ocean lover, has set up a project titled 'Like Water' to explore innovative ways to reconnect with who we are, our environment and each other through water. Interesting work, I salute you for it!!

What does this Ocean-Blue Connection Feel Like?

To address this question, I am choosing 3 different time frames to describe my personal experience of sea-swimming over the last 8 months.

January 2021

Our first day. It's freezing cold as we change into our swimming gear. Relucent to remove my warm jacket. I pause. I think, "Oh this is pure madness"!! But there are 3 of us, egging one another on. The banter. Fun and laughter. Some swearing too!!. No wetsuits, we battle the path to the waters. I glance at the steps into the ocean and decide, heck, let's jump. This was my first experience of very cold water swimming and I was unprepared for the sudden shock to the system that occurred as my body plunged into the sea. A deep intake of breath. The utter sensation of cold. Hand and feet numb within seconds. I notice my breathing increases. As a Mindfulness teacher and nurse, I am fascinated. I focus on my breath. Slowly it settles. I am so in my physical body right now. No space for thoughts or worries. Just survival. I begin to swim, staying close to the Blackrock tower area. I am getting cold. Checking how my 2 swim buddies are, we are all beginning to get cold. We decide to exit. Quickly changing into warm clothes, I feel a sudden, deep calm. My hands begin to shake as we drink hot tea and soup. Feeling good, we part company. I drive home. Warm shower and I am astonished at two things that occur. Firstly, emotionally, I feel fantastic, calm and on a high. Like the afterglow of intimacy. Totally immersive. Totally connected. Secondly, within a few hours, I am exhausted. And sleep so soundly that night.

I think of Wim Hof, The Ice Man who I admire and am an avid fan on social media. I read his books to try to understand what has occurred physiologically and why the extraordinary elation on coming out of the sea that lasted many hours afterwards.

Wim Hof (2020: 33) explains that "The cold goes past the mind, past the conditioning, past all comfort-zone behaviourism, past our weakness to make us strong". Cold water stimulates the vagus nerve, which runs from the neck to the abdomen and is in charge of turning off the 'fight, flight or freeze' stress response of the body. If we have high vagus tone our parasympathetic nervous system is working and our bodies relax faster after stress. In addition, cold water swimming increases the heart rate. Our bodies respond by releasing a protein called brain derived neurotrophic factor (BDNF). This helps protect and repair our memory neurons. At the same time, our bodies realise endorphins which block the discomfort of the cold and make us feel euphoric. I find it interesting to understand how our bodies react and adapt to sea swimming, certainly a resiliency enhancing experience.

February 2021

A different day. Blustery and cold. Wind howling. Hailstones hitting our bodies with force. We banter and laugh. In we go. Jump!! Wow! This is new. It's cold, but we are more used to the cold now and it no longer bothers us as much as when we started. Our bodies have adjusted. A little anyway!! But swimming in hailstones. That is a first. It's totally exhilarating. The hailstones dancing shamanic patterns on the water. The sheer joy of being there. The marvel of it. The excitement of it. We laugh. Like children. So happy, excited to have caught this moment. Rare and beautiful. We don't feel cold. We swim, chat, laugh, thread water and generally take in the landscape, the dark clouds, the rolling mountains barely visible in the distance. Our connection. Bonded by laugher and fun in this strange and wonderful moment of utter happiness. We marvel at our courage, congratulate ourselves for our bravery. Our self-esteem is high, our sense of achievement overwhelming, our commitment to one another and to our daily swim acknowledged. We are feeling emotionally happy, mentally strong, physically good. What a day, one that will live forever, in our nostalgic memory pool for years to come.

July 2021

High tide. Water is now warm, no longer challenging us physiologically with the cold. We have grown used to sea swimming, the water is calm and the sky is blue. We decide to swim further, stretching our physical fitness a little more. The water is full, it's a strange sensation, like a bowl. Cradling my body, protecting me, keeping me warm. I'm enjoying this totally immersive experience. The light rays reflecting the water. Shimmering. I lie on my back. Watch the sky. Swimming. Silently, quietly along. Clouds and blue sky passing me by. Catching sounds. The gentle ripple of the waves. The excited shriek of children on the nearby beach. I feel I am everything and nothing. No worries, no cares. Blissful oblivion!

Sea swimming for the last 8 months has been an incredible time for me. I have experienced a very deep sense of connectedness to myself, my SwimPod3 and the wider seascape. It has been emotionally exhilarating, mentally restorative, physically demanding at times, but always spiritually special. It is totally immersive and wonderful. I cod you not, I will continue....

Conclusion

There is a lovely phrase the Japanese use called 'living water' which means that we humans pour some of ourselves into the water when we get into it. It, in turn, somehow takes our emotions and reconfigures them, it takes our physical aches and our mental anguish and soothes and calms them. In this way the water is not just alive with its own ecosystem, it is also alive with us and our emotions. I can vouch for this experience as it explains the multi-layered connectedness I feel in and with the water. It is totally immersive, challenging, fun, beautiful, freeing, its connectedness goes deep into my heart, my inner being and my soul. It allows solitude and silence that forges a connectedness to presence that goes deep. In the words of Gordon Hempton:

'Silence is not the absence of something, but the presence of everything'

Nuggets for Millennials

- Solitude
- Find a place of quiet that you enjoy
- Just sit
- Be silent
- Bring awareness to the breath in your body
- Listen to the sound around you
- See the sights around you
- Let yourself go into a space of wonder
- Be not afraid
- Be at peace.

*Cautionary Note: If you are going to try sea-swimming, why not try it in the summer time and gradually build up your stamina for the winter. Never swim alone. Know the limits of your body. Do not swim out of your depth. Wear appropriate swim gear, wetsuit, boots, gloves and a visible hat in winter. Take heed of weather condition, advice from the lifeguards, and other signs telling of rip currents and water conditions. Join a swimming club and be guided by more experienced members. Enjoy!

References

Barry Harry (2018) Emotional Resilience: How to Safeguard your Mental Health. Great Britain: Orion Spring Publishing.

Bauman Z. (2002) *Liquid Modernity*. Cambridge, UK: Polity Press.

Beck U. (2005) *Risk Society: Towards a New Modernity*. London: Sage Publication.

Britton E. & Kindermann G. & Domegan C. & Carlin C. (2020) Blue care: a systematic reivew of blue space interventions for health and well-being. *Health Promotion International*. 35(1), 50-69.

Carney S. (2019) *What Doesn't Kill Us*. London: Scribe Publication.

Coplan R. & Bowker J. (2014) All Alone: Multiple Perspectives on the Study of Solitude. In: Coplan R & Bowker (Eds) *The Handbook of Solitude: Psychological Perspectives on Social Isolation, Social Withdrawal and the Experience of Being Alone*. New York: Wiley-Blackwell. 3-13.

Crane B. (2017) The Virtues of Isolation. The Psychological Benefits of Being Alone. *The Atlantic*. Available at: https://www.theatlantic.com/health/archive/2017/03/the-virtues-of-isolation/521100/ Accessed on 24/07/2021

Deloitte Global Millennial and Generation Z Survey Report (2021) Available at: www.Deloitte.com/millennialssurvey 2021 Accessed on: 25/07/2021

Delmar N. (2018) Generation Panic. Why is there so much anxiety among Millennials. *The Irish Times Monday June 11, 2018*. Available at: https://www.irishtimes.com/life-and-style/health-family/generation-panic-why-is-there-so-much-anxiety-among-millennials-1.3521341 Accessed on: 22/07/2021.

Gennep A. (1960) *The Rites of Passage*. Chicago: University of Chicago.

Hof W. (2020) The Wim Hof Method. Activate Your Potential, Transcend Your Limits. London: Ebury Publishing.

Kelly C. (2021) Blue Spaces: How and Why Water Can Make You Feel Better. London: Welbeck Balance.

Larson R. W. (1990) The solitary side of life. An examination of the time people spend alone from childhood to old age. *Developmental Review*. 10, 155-183

Merton T. (1958) *Thoughts in Solitude*. London: MacMillan Publication.

Naor L. & Mayseless O. (2020) The wilderness solo experience: A unique practice of silence and solitude for personal growth. *Frontiers in Psychology. Review.* 11(547067) 1-15.

Nguyen T. & Ryan R. M. & Deci E. L. (2017) Solitude as an Approach to Affective Self-Regulation. *Personality and Social Psychology Bulletin.* 1-15.

Noone P. (2019) Finding Your Signature Strength. In: Mac Giolla Bhui & Noone P. (Eds) *Mental Health for Millennials.* 3, 4-16.

Resilience and the Sea:
Why I have Embraced the Open Waters during the Global Pandemic

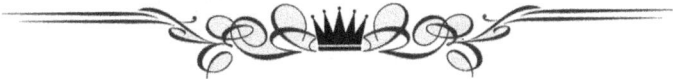

Cliona Beirne

Introduction

I'm a twenty-five-year-old millennial living just a twenty minute walk to the ocean in Galway, Ireland. And the ocean is where I've been spending quite a bit of time these past eight months. Swimming. Deep breathing. Living. And it's exhilarating. It's resilience in every sense of the word because in the sea, I bounce back from my working day. I use this time in the deep water to feel alive, to appreciate nature and what is important to me.

Challenges and Stresses as a Millennial

A study conducted by Maynooth University Professor Audra Mockaitis (2020) states that millennials are showing lower levels of wellbeing, due primarily to the COVID-19 pandemic and the government imposed emphasis on staff remote working. Even though we millennials live in a constantly connected bubble of social media and the next big hashtag or trending, Professor Mockaitis (2020) states that we struggled far more than the generation before us, Baby Boomers. I believe this is because we are so busy trying to be accepted that we do not know what it is like to survive as a single unit, without the potential judgement of our peers.

The lack of routine and structure from having to work at home has caused burnout of our mental health. Once surrounded by our friends in work, pubs, restaurants, our homes, have now become complete isolation for all too many millennials. A stark realisation of what the norm became for many of us - bed, kitchen, work area at home, kitchen, living room, bed. Something we are not used to and have never been exposed to is a very unwelcome loneliness. Thankfully, during the pandemic, I was counted as direct labour or frontline where we had to be in our physical working environment to complete the job responsibilities allocated. This stabilised some elements of peer interaction, much like our soon-to-be-formed swim pod where in the latest lockdown in January 2021 we began meeting up.

Why I Started Sea Swimming

Our sea swim pod became a foundation, just like a house needs to remain a solid structure. I needed to ensure that my foundation was more grounded than ever. Sea swimming brings many benefits both mentally and physically. Once you are in the water your survival mode kicks in-fight or flight, your body hits the winter waters, a cold surge overpowers your body and breathing becomes minimal, but you adapt overtime by fighting the urge to fail.

I started sea swimming because the gyms were closed, and it was something I found very hard to adapt to without the gym. I normally use the gym as my mental health 'time out' and to feel physically good after completing a workout. Without it I felt I had no structure to my evenings, not exercising at all and I needed some motivation. Sea swimming in winter gives a heightened adrenaline rush which has a profound effect on your body and mind (Patrick Kelleher, 2019) and this interested me as I love a challenge. The release of endorphins and serotonin even after five to ten minutes in the water has enough resiliency to withhold in the body all day (Hof, 2020). Sea swimming proved to me, psychologically, that you can overcome something which initially felt impossible and overwhelming.

How Sea Swimming has Helped my Mental Health and Resiliency

A quote on resiliency which resonates with me and often gives me pause to reflect.is,

"The strongest oak of the forest is not the one that is protected from the storm and hidden from the sun. It's the one that stands in the open where it is compelled to struggle for its existence against the winds and rains and the scorching sun" (www.actorsmotivation.com 2012)

Just like the oak tree, our swim pods similarities are highlighted through our strengths and resistance to allowing our collective and individual mental health to collapse in such uncertain times. The swim pod meet up at least three times a week, mentally solidifying that a routine was established - something us as humans crave.

With the whirlwind of uncertainties that each of us faced, at least we knew that meeting up was our time out to enjoy each other's company. Each of us grasped to one another's strengths whilst also joking about something silly someone else iterated. This was the balance that the swim pod brought, where outside disturbance was kept to a minimum and being present became the core focus of our group. Sea swimming has enabled me to conquer a new personal accomplishment. The dependency on finding a new more resilient version of myself was being able to complete daily sea swimming regardless of the weather conditions. This shows, the true power of mental strength and how you can push it far enough to alter your mood and thought process in a positive way. Throwing yourself into the icy cold Atlantic waters of Galway Bay brings upon new levels of intrinsic satisfaction through this sense of euphoria from within. A sense of completion, a sense of belonging to the swim pod group that push each other to be stronger versions of ourselves. In our group of three there is unity.

References

Napoleon hill. (2012). Resiliency. Available: https://actorsmotivation.wordpress.com/. Last accessed 30th of July 2021.

Prof Audra Mockaitis. (2020). Millennials experience most difficulties coping with Covid-19 workplace disruptions. Available: https://www.maynoothuniversity.ie/research/maynoothworks/news-events/latest-news/millennials-experience-most-difficulties-coping-covid-19-workplace-disruptions. Last accessed 01st August 2021.

Patrick Kelleher. (2019). The addictive magic of swimming in the sea in winter: 'It's life affirming'. Available: https://www.irishtimes.com/life-and-style/the-addictive-magic-of-swimming-in-the-sea-in-winter-it-s-life-affirming-1.4074180. Last accessed 01st August 2021.

On Resiliency

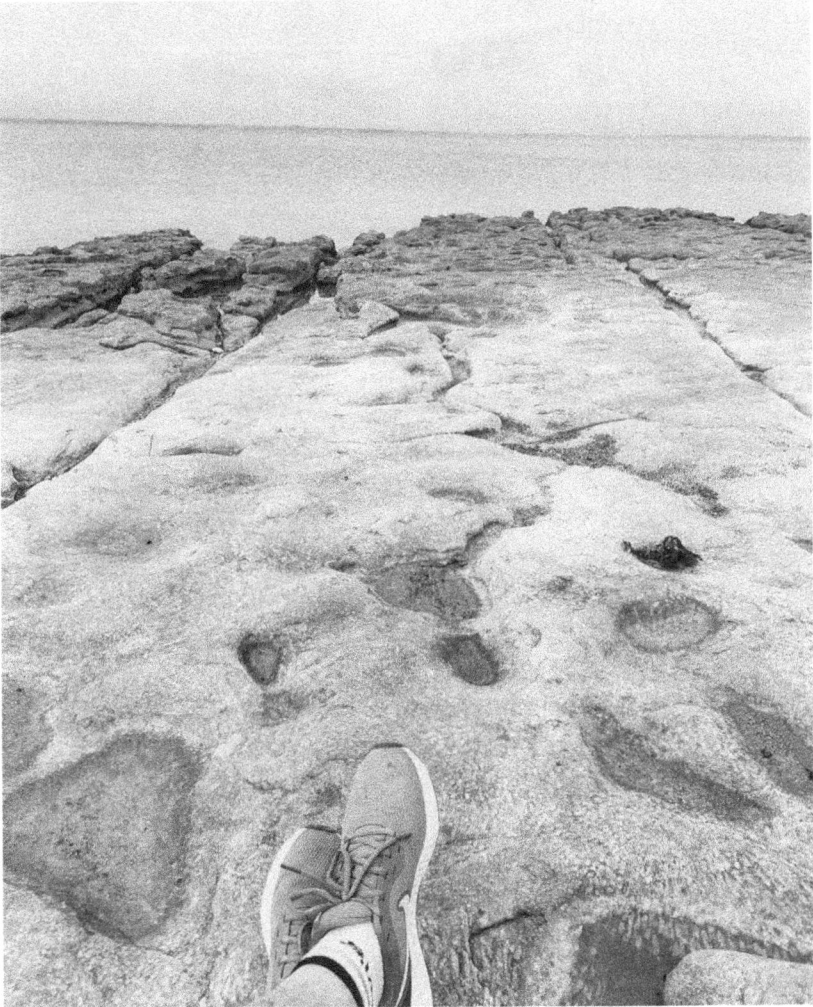

'You Are Resilience'

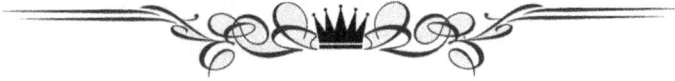

Dr. Mary Helen Hensley

If the publisher had not given a specified word-count for each submission for this book, my contribution would have been complete in three words:

You Are Resilience

The world as we knew it, only a few short years ago, has deconstructed, abolishing antiquated ideas, demanding a more conscious and inclusive dialogue from the ever-growing numbers that command our attention across all platforms of social media and society. We humans have undergone a metamorphosis of sorts, reconstructing the way we conduct ourselves in person, in cyber-space and within the confines of our own homes. Throw a global pandemic in for good measure; lockdowns, social distancing, mask- wearing out of fear of contracting some mysterious ailment lurking in the tiny droplets of your neighbour's breath, and suddenly, yesterday's three-piece Ted Baker suit has been replaced by a crumpled shirt and tie, with boxers and bare feet, invisible just below the "Zoom line".

Traditionally, we have defined resilience as strength, tenacity or the ability to bounce back from difficult situations. After the last two years we've all put in, I'd like to throw another adjective in to the mix; adaptability.

What is in your own personal constitution that puts you amongst those who are still here, still with us, able to read these words? Tragically, we all have lost or know someone who has lost a family member or friend, to old age, disease, an accident, or suicide. In the last two years, we have been inundated with a staggering number of losses attributed to the pandemic for a variety of reasons... not simply due to a virus. We have also seen an unprecedented number of individuals struggling with their mental health. There are those who fell in to this great global pause already enduring serious stress. There is also a new group of individuals who would have never thought that the words, "I think I might be depressed" or "I think I might need help", would ever come out of their mouths *in a million years*. An incredible number of observers were suddenly experiencers. And then, another new wave began to swell.

As people worried about childcare, graduating college, paying mortgages, buying groceries, providing for their families, all because they had no idea when they would return to normal or receive a paycheck again, a new category of stress saw a massive rise in its ranks. Not necessarily struggling with something clinical or with a label, but still under a huge amount of fresh angst, many people found themselves barely keeping their heads above water, whilst attempting to deal with the daily, ongoing issues of a loved one with serious mental health concerns. You might be the one they were dealing with, or you might be the one who found yourself desperately clinging to your own sanity, while attempting to preserve it for someone you love.

Again, I ask... why are you still standing? I bet you never would have thought that your resilience, your adaptability, all boils down to *managing your food.*

Seriously? Food? Yes, food. The population at large has recently watched the 3D world around them, blow right past 4D and into a 5D world where animated avatars and bank PINs carry as much weight as a real flesh and blood humans. For years I have been explaining a concept to audiences that is now becoming tangible.

Everything is food.

The traditional definition of food as any substance consumed to provide nutritional support for an organism just doesn't cut it in a 5D world, where the fifth element is choice. Food is now redefined as that which is consumed by both body and mind, therefore affecting change in the physical and emotional states. Every single day, you have an infinite number of choices to make about the 'food' with which you will feed yourself. From the decision to properly hydrate, to the choice between fresh or processed meats and veg, to stimulants such as caffeine or nicotine or harder drugs that can lift you up or bring you down. Will you listen to a humorous podcast on the way to work or sit home and flick through endless debates over Covid protocols in your newsfeed? Will you feed your mind with a gossip session on Snapchat or pop in the air pods to deter anyone from attempting to actually interact with you whilst sitting on the bus? Each and every one of these things becomes the daily diet, the lifestyle choices that will determine your experience of resilience to the world around you.

Taking some time to power down, kick back and have a real heart to heart *with yourself* about what sort of *food* is on your personal menu these days, is an easy, yet powerful way of strengthening your ability to bounce back from pandemonium, real worries or anxiety-induced paper dragons. Resilience isn't something that just happens on demand, like a sudden burst of adrenaline-fueled energy that allows a mother to lift a tremendous weight off of her injured child. Resilience is a slow burn. For some, it is best acquired with a daily diet of positive stimulus, healthy meals, time outdoors, up-lifting conversations with friends or a challenging, yet rewarding day at work. For others, surrounding themselves with mood music, writing the dark musings of their hearts, hours on end with a remote control in hand killing zombies, feeding the addiction to drama with thumbs that can text at one hundred words a minute… for these folks, resilience might show up in ripped up fish nets, a trench coat and ink black nails. When judgement is pushed aside over the 'right' way to survive in this crazy world, we become acutely aware that our personal definitions of tenacity and resilience are as numerous *and brilliant* as the stars on a mid-summer's night.

If you are reading this, YOU ARE RESILENCE. If you've made it through the last two years by the skin of your teeth, the proverbial seat of your pants…YOU ARE RESILENCE. If you moved to the safety of your childhood home, if you moved away from home, if you met a new love, if you ended a difficult relationship, if you started a new job, if you had the courage to leave a job you couldn't stand…YOU ARE RESILIENCE. If you spent late nights at the drive-thru, indulging your cravings, if you lost a few pounds, if you started running again, if you gave your body a much-needed break, if your circle of friends looks nothing like it used to, if you clung to the steadfast companions of your youth, if you started a new course, if you stopped spending time and money on a project that no longer serves you…YOU ARE RESILIENCE. If you wrote your first song, your first line of poetry, if you started to meditate or if you sat quietly on the couch in your own company for hours on end…YOU ARE RESILIENCE. If your fingers are stained with the paint from a new piece of art you created, if you kept that one little cactus alive, if you sent a text a friend just to check on them, if you asked for help, or gave help to someone in need… YOU ARE RESILIENCE. If you cried, if you laughed, if you sang at the top of your lungs, if you played games, read all of the self-help books, if you thought about ending it all, but didn't…YOU ARE RESILIENCE.

It doesn't matter how you've spent your time, how your mind raced, how you couldn't seem to cling to a single coherent thought, how brilliant or productive you've been, how many days in a row you wore the same pyjamas, who you made proud or who was disappointed in your choices… you've made it to right here, right now, this very moment. You owe no one an explanation, because messy or beautiful, harrowing or with grace and ease, you adapted the very best way you knew how and you showed up….and that, my friends, IS the definition of RESILIENCE.

RESILIENCE -
Our Invisible Fabric of Resistance

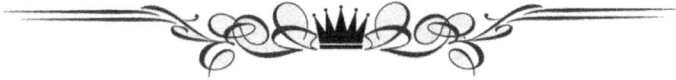

Renée Sigel

In the social mythology of 'strength versus weakness', we are raised to believe in many negative artificial constructs which shape our sense of who we are, versus who we should, or even, wish to become. This social dynamic begins to play itself out from the moment, as toddlers, we start stepping out into life and begin interacting with others. Traits like reticence, confidence, introversion, extroversion, brattiness, generosity, empathy, disinterest, whether predicated at that early age by precarity or wealth, or not, take shape in these very early encounters. Much is written about "nature versus nurture" and already at kindergarten, stereotypical characterisations tend to be assigned, often dangerously so, without much forethought as to the deeper implications this kind of psychological pigeonholing can have on developing self- esteem.

The Nature of Brain Architecture

The architecture of the brain is constructed from a continual process of developing connectivity between individual neurons; simple skills form

37

in the womb and from birth, the proliferation of neural connectivity becomes increasingly complex. During the first few years of infancy, it is estimated that over a million neural connections are made every second. In time this process slows, and certain connections are naturally 'pruned' to maximise the efficiency of brain circuitry. While this a dynamic, rather than a static chemical process enabling a multiplicity of cognitive and motor skills across all areas of the brain, for which natural aptitude, talent or artistry also emerges, it has been shown that the 'quality' of these formative connective neural processes creates a foundation from which all other developmental connections then follow. It is a relatively recent discovery that experience fundamentally influences how genes interact, which by turn shapes the qualitative or 'neglectful'/ negative development of brain architecture. Genes are the blueprint for brain circuitry, but that is not where their influence ends. The fact that individual experiences directly influence how genes are turned on or off, technically termed 'how geneses are expressed - (how readable they might be at a cellular level) - pretty much makes a moot point of the old dictum about nature or nurture, with respect to how and who the child grows into being as an individual. It also accounts for the vastly different traits and divergent 'innate skillsets' in siblings can be even though raised in the same household.

Children, especially toddlers are like sponges and absorb everything they experience around them. It is known now, through genetic and neurological research that neither the brain, nor human nature is pre-determined by immutable genetic coding; rather, the architecture of the brain is constantly evolving through a process of *neural epigenetic modification*, or developmental processes termed 'serve and return' and that genes respond to experience.

The Shaping of "I"

So, if genetic markers we inherit are not immutable but changeable through the experiences from the youngest age, just how does what we experience influence the shaping of our cerebral architecture, making us who we are, or could become?

Epigenetic research so far shows that our neural circuitry, once created are reinforced and strengthened through repeated use. This does not however make them immune to the chemical changes which are triggered as a result of positive or negative experiences. Genes respond to experiences because all learning occurs experientially. Genes respond chemically as epigenetic markers within each gene trigger not only how much protein is made by the gene, but also where in the gene; it is known that typically such genetic alterations tend to occur in exactly those cells which can compromise organ functionality. The impact experiential changes have on the development of specialized organs, especially during early years of a child's development can have a drastic impact on the physical as well as mental health over a lifetime.

Experiential development in a young child necessitates a process of what is termed 'serve and return'; i.e., positive, or negative reinforcement in the responses an infant, toddler or even teen receives from parental figures or caregivers. The absence of responsive care, which is essentially neglectful, unreliable, or disinterested care creates the 'difficult, unresponsive or delinquent' child. A dysfunctional human being is not self-made, even in adulthood, trauma, violence, assault, brutality fundamentally changes the character of a person and now we can understand how this occurs at a genetic level; genes and experiences work intrinsically to construct, modify, or utterly alter brain architecture.

Researchers are beginning to understand that genes are not only responsive to 'toxic stress', they are also susceptible to nutritional, emotional and psychological issues which result from these deeply disruptive kinds of 'serves and returns' which are created through trauma.

As explained in this Harvard University article:

Experiences Affect How Genes Are Expressed

Inside the nucleus of each cell in our bodies, we have **chromosomes**, which contain the code for characteristics that pass to the next generation. Within these chromosomes, specific segments of genetic code, known as **genes,** make up long, double-helix strands of DNA.

Experiences leave a chemical "signature" on genes that determines whether and how genes are expressed.

Children inherit approximately 23,000 genes from their parents, but not every gene does what it was designed to do. Experiences leave a chemical "signature" on genes that determines whether and how the genes are expressed. Collectively, those signatures are called the **epigenome.**

The brain is particularly responsive to experiences and environments during early development. **External experiences** spark signals between neurons, which respond by producing proteins. These **gene regulatory proteins** head to the nucleus of the neural cell, where they either attract or repel enzymes that can attach them to the genes. Positive experiences, such as exposure to rich learning opportunities, and negative influences, such as malnutrition or environmental toxins, can change the chemistry that encodes genes in brain cells — a change that can be temporary or permanent. This process is called epigenetic modification. (1)

What makes this new kind of study revelatory is that we no longer need to feel that we are somehow at fault for being "less than", "weak" or worst, "unworthy"…

Our Invisible Fabric of Resistance

In the ever burgeoning 'wellness sector', positivity is being sold as a fundamental principle to inner balance and overall mental health. This has opened the field of wellness to a proliferation of amateur 'expertise' in all manner of approaches and skillsets pertaining to creating and even 'enhancing' resilience in the face of 'uncertainty' and whatever set of 'complex issues' are sold as the challenges pertaining to a given resiliency sales pitch. Lists abound declaring the habits and or characteristics of the resilient mind and these 'experts' then go on to espouse ways in which you too can initiate, or enhance your own resiliency, taken on the assumption that you're reading their offers of courses because you do not feel resilient at all.

These kinds of 'wellness gurus' feed off very dangerous misconceptions essentially based in an overriding general ignorance of the subject about which they claim expertise. So, what is resilience?

In purely scientific terms when looking at materials, resilience is defined as the material's capacity to absorb energy to its limit of elasticity and to release that energy without it creating a permanent distortion. In terms of measuring and proving resilience of a given material a modulus of resilience, measured in a joule per cubic meter is calculated as maximum energy by measuring the material displacement of the yield strain curve from zero to the elastic limit and ascertaining strength under strain to gauge the toughness – resilience of the material without distortion or permanent damage once that energy or pressure is released.

We can look at human resilience in the same way. Our genes respond to human experiences meaning that like any other material its absorption of negative or positive energy, from enriching, affirming reciprocal relationships to neglect, abuse and traumatic experiences will shift and shape the kind of proteins our genes produce and define the maximum absorption before permanent damage or distortion occurs. The difference is, we measure resilience, failure, toughness, weakness, and strength as attributes and think about them in emotional terms, thereby shaping our opinion of ourselves and others by these very limited categorical values.

Within this context, resilience is a field of increasing scientific study, not only in the scientific context of matter, or physiological or eco-systems, but at an epigenic level too. It is a new area of research and caution abounds in terms of the claims that can made as to how and why, among humans, resilience seems to come naturally to some and not others.

In a research paper on the *psychobiology and molecular genetics of resilience*, published in Neuroscience in 2009, the researchers aim was to *"…outline and attempt to integrate recent developments in resilience research from psychosocial, developmental, genetic and neurobiological perspectives."* (2)

The paper highlighted that examining stress responses at 'multiple phenotypic levels' has shown

"… Numerous hormones, neurotransmitters and neuropeptides are involved in the acute psychobiological responses to stress. Differences in the function, balance and interaction of these factors underlie inter-individual variability in stress resilience."

This kind of detailed molecular, genetic, and neural study has been made possible by advances in both scientific and technological advances and

"… suggest that genetic influences on biological responses — such as neural responses to affective stimuli, measured with brain imaging — are larger than genetic influences on complex behavioural responses."

This paper points further to the likelihood that,

"Examining stress responses at multiple phenotypic levels, including not only behavioural and psychological measurements, but also measurements of neurochemical, neuroendocrine and neural systems, could thus help to delineate an integrative model of resilience."

All of which would go a long way to informing mental health clinicians of deeper causes for behavioural outcomes and very likely lead to different, perhaps more appropriate treatments for depression, PTSD and long-term effects of trauma. None of this deeper epigenetic research seeks to undermine previous and current research and emphasis on psychosocial determinants of resilience to stress, if anything, it broadens the scope of intervention and recovery, if for no other reason that it kicks the generalisation of weak-versus-strong character/ personality, in the booty, for good.

More importantly, what this means throughout childhood into our adult lives, in the scope of all our "experiences", is that we are not necessarily 'doomed' to be or to feel victimised, nor destined to be held hostage by the anxiety that might occur from negative experiences. Healing too can alter the gene regulatory proteins and so change the encoding chemistry in our brain cells, dramatically altering how we feel and relate to the world around us. It means we can and do heal from traumatic past-experience.

I was invited to write this chapter because of my own 'extreme life experiences' and to share my views on resiliency. I felt it remiss not to first share facts about how we are shaped by experience and to highlight that our genetic mapping continues to shift and alter throughout our lives. What I have learnt is that we do have the power to shift our response to whatever might happen to us. How we believe in something or the extent to which we buy into doubt, whether construed by others, or contrived by our own negative mindset at any given moment, plays a fundamental role in whether we become the victim or hero of our own story. This sounds flippant perhaps on first reading, but it is everything but: After a lifetime of traumatic experiences, more loss than I care to recount, and decades of intense sadness, self-loathing, and mostly shame, I am finally stepping out into a life of my own making.

Renée Sigel

I don't usually share details of my life story publicly. In writing this piece however, I realise it would be disingenuous to write it without sharing with you, the reader, something of the kind of traumatizing landscape I've negotiated since childhood. Context, as they say is everything.

I was raised in an era when children were *'seen and not heard'*. Obedience and compliance were the mainstay of one's upbringing. As a child you have no voice, no actual presence that is an engaged expression of self, wherein the 'serve and return' scientists speak of in the building of brain architecture is so vital, rather, you realise yourself as an attentive, obliging, yet ostensibly passive entity, navigating a wholly unpredictable landscape of adults. Your objective is not to incur their wrath and or punishment and yet you know this is never achievable. Your transgressions are inevitable. And much of what you do in your childhood is between dare and suppliance, driven by needs of visceral self-expression and survival.

At the age of three, when a supposed 'caregiver', a Catholic nun, no less, takes it upon herself to physical threaten your life by pressing a pillow over your head so that you will comply to her command for your silence, you realise very, very quickly you're on your own. Your mother is on the other side of the world on honeymoon and left you at a nunnery, in the care of tyranny. No one is coming to fetch you: You resolve to taking care of yourself and never asking anyone for anything, ever. And so it begins.

By the age of six you're adopted, later discovering your biological father gave you up legally and emotionally. You're reminded daily that you're adopted and of your duty to gratitude, obedience, and silence, for anything but might ruin the marriage and it would then be all your fault. You take to dancing on the driveway imitating the ballet class you watch across the road through their wall-lined mirrors until the teacher convinces your mother to let you start lessons. You thrive in dance class. By the time you're nine, your dad's lungs collapse, and the drinking worsens once he returns from hospital.

Your sister has become your nemesis and you take to hiding in trees for hours to test if anyone realizes your missing. No one does.

One Sunday morning you're woken by yelling and screaming. You open your bedroom door to find your mother crawling along the corridor in pain while your dad stands over with a riding crop whipping her and yelling that she won't get away with trying to get rid of him. She orders you to run and get the neighbour, a medical doctor; you scramble in blind panic and come back breathless keeping a distance from the chaos inside your home. You watch your mother carried off on a stretcher in an ambulance and you rage inside at them both. No one tells you or your sister what is happening, until days later: Cancer. She needs an operation and then cobalt and radiation treatment. No hospital visits for children allowed.

Once she is home, you become her companion and confidante. She takes you along to all her treatments. You watch her suffer the side effects; she loses weight and all her hair. You help her select wigs. She goes into remission. Dad's drinking worsens. They seem to stop being friends. Fights become more frequent. Mum seems to sleep all the time. Lithium and Valium. One day you lose it: You hear voices, want to flee, curl up in a ball and tear off your skin, all at the same time. A doctor is called, and you're pinned to the bed and given an intravenous sedative. You lose two days to sleep and hallucinations. You wake up and can barely remember anything but yelling while being pinned to the bed and the needle. You're fed chicken noodle soup and told to go and play. No one asks if you are okay.

Several years later, you meet a boy and you're infatuated by his artistry. After months of casual dating, he asks you to be his girlfriend. It is the night his best friend commits suicide, and his father dies from a heart attack. Three months later, it's January 2nd, you bicker with your mother and she leaves for work really upset. You promise to wait up for her to come home, to make it up to her. Only she doesn't. You never see her again. In the early hours the phone rings; there's been an accident. The ambulance on which she is a paramedic was hit by a drunken driver in an intersection. She's thrust across the intersection and the ambulance rolls. She is in emergency surgery. Doctors trying to save her life. Your rouse your father and you all head to the hospital, in shock.

In the ER you sit next to a sobbing, drunken middle- aged man in a suit, with a few bruises. You find out later he was the driver. You sit at the funeral wondering at the world of strangers who all seemed to know your mother and you, none of them. Two days later you turn 20 and for the rest of your life that birthday remains a blank. No one asks how you are doing. You and the boy bond over loss and call it love. It is the start of a different nightmare.

You leave home, move in together for a while it feels and is 'perfect'. The cracks appear slowly at first and you ignore them, convincing yourself you're imagining things. Then comes the medical diagnosis which explains the spells of involuntary paralysis he experiences. Little can be done. Everything shifts. He denigrates and shames you, has you 'serve' his career lessening the time you have to commit to your own. Threats begin. The violence is discreet at first. You try and talk to people; no one is listening, no takes you seriously. You're surely the one to be exaggerating. You decide to study for a degree, enroll at Uni and work part time to pay your way. You go back to dance and are offered a studio of a major dance figure. You're laughed at when you share the news. You don't go back. You disappear into work and writing. You get your degree, have your first poetry seriously published in an academic journal. You are commissioned to edit your first book anthology for a university department. You go on to get a job in an art gallery and begin collaborating with a well-known artist. You freelance with the national newspaper and various magazines. The relationship becomes increasingly toxic. You still don't leave. You're determined none of it will get the better of you. You ignore the fact it might be: You're taking care of your father who is in and out of drying out clinics and eventually is handed a suspended sentence for driving under the influence. He is increasingly belligerent, and you stop seeing him.

You get a call in the middle of the night; a friend has been fatally stabbed at his restaurant. A few weeks later, another friend, strangled during a robbery at her home. Then you escape two bomb blasts by the skin of your teeth. You find yourself one morning in town on the way to the city library when a street battle breaks out between police and demonstrators and you're caught in the crossfire; you scramble to protect a young boy selling oranges and he dies beneath your body and you see his mother drop as she calls out his name; and somehow, you get to walk away. You can't shop shaking for days, you don't sleep. You say nothing. It occurs to no one to ask you how you are. Weeks later you're inadvertently caught up in student demonstrations on campus, you're among the women beaten with batons and are forced to watch as riot police set their dogs loose on students. The scenes haunt your sleep.

Six months after your daughter is born, you're offered a weekend away 'to save the marriage'. You are taken to your favourite place. There you are raped at knife point and told he owns you now in every way. All you know how to do is shut down into silence. You loathe yourself more than ever; even more than you loathe him. You want to scream but dissociate instead: you stop feeling, you stop yourself from being a woman anymore. You slip into the mechanics of it all. Feel nothing.

At some point the phone rings in the early hours. You let it ring. You know it is about your father. He'd been mugged the week before drawing cash at a shopping centre. Strangers found him lying in a pool of blood between parked cars. He died that night from pneumonia.

Renée Sigel

Two years later, the secret service turns up at your home with an ultimatum, which you cannot accept. You're accused of treason for wanting to change the status quo. You refuse and within weeks, your life is being shut down. Bank account closed. House seized. And you leave with nothing but a suitcase, a trunk of soft toys and 120 bucks in your pocket to start a life on the other side of the world.

On the other side of the world, you find yourself in a new country with the father of your child and your spousal rapist in need of a kidney transplant. You become his nurse. You work nights. His ex-sister-in law turns out to be a match and she donates a kidney. Surgery is difficult and the organ is rejected, and the operation needs to be redone. He barely survives intensive care.

He recovers some degree of health and starts an affair. You file for divorce. That same week you get a call; a long-time friend has been murdered by her boyfriend; he'd threatened it for years and finally did it – came home one lunch time and stabbed her fourteen times. You want to tear your hair out. Scream yell, go mental. No one asks how if you're okay.

Your daughter bonds with a young man and soon you're flat sharing to ease her experience of the divorce. You marry again and have another two daughters. You move to Italy to give your eldest the chance of her own life. You find yourself alone in a new country raising three young children. You try and make friends. You make one. A close friend as it turns out, only she commits suicide two days before her own son's eleventh birthday. All you can do is retreat from everything and everyone. You feel your body caving, you're falling ill. No one believes you.

You barely muster your way through the days. Your insomnia is extreme; you burn and crash, lose hours in a day and you cannot fathom how. Anger builds. Your ex dies and cassette tapes surface. You discover you were set up all along. The tapes are proof. You want nothing more than to lose your sh*t … but you don't even know how anymore. So, you stay silent.

You raise three daughters over a decade pretty much on your own. You work relentlessly to try and earn a meagre living; nothing works. You just keep at it driven by an inexplicable stubbornness, even in the face of blatant disinterest which has your soul feel like it's drowning in a desert.

You publish books and a magazine. You start up a lifestyle deign company and are embraced by fashion professionals in Paris. It feels like you can take on the world. You try. Everything just burns instead.

It's over a decade later and you're moving to a new country again. This time things will be different. And they are. You fall while walking the dog and break your ankle. And so, begins a seven year stretch of eight surgical procedures and learning to walk from scratch. And you'd think trauma would have had its day by now. No such luck . . .

I've been told I'm the most resilient of people, by friends, colleagues and even strangers, on occasion: I can tell you quite honestly, I wouldn't begin to know what that feels like. All I can say about "being resilient", from my own personal experience, is that no matter what kind of behaviour people felt entitled to enforce on me, subject me to, or traumatic events I witnessed which were out of my control, for however crushed and bruised my soul and psyche felt, or for the existential threat that I know is still there and very real, I've only known one thing for certain, I refuse to be broken.

Is this resilience? I have no idea; perhaps. If it means I have a epigenome to thank for it, I am ever more appreciative, though, that from which it does not keep me immune, is the trauma itself. Having worked through the self-loathing, the sadness, and the shame, most especially the shame, I still must step inside all of the trauma, internalized over a lifetime and more than anything, I will have to trust my refusal to broken, that immersion into it, will not break me in the end.

Renée Sigel

References

(1) Centre on The Developing Child, Harvard University.
https://developingchild.harvard.edu/science/key-concepts/brain-architecture/

(2) Psychobiology and Molecular Genetics of Resilience. *A Feder, E.J.Nestler, D.S.Charney*, published in Nature reviews. Neuroscience, 01 Jun 2009, 10(6):446-457 DOI: 10.1038/nrn2649 PMID: 19455174 PMCID: PMC2833107 / http://europepmc.org/article/MED/194551

Nature is Resilience

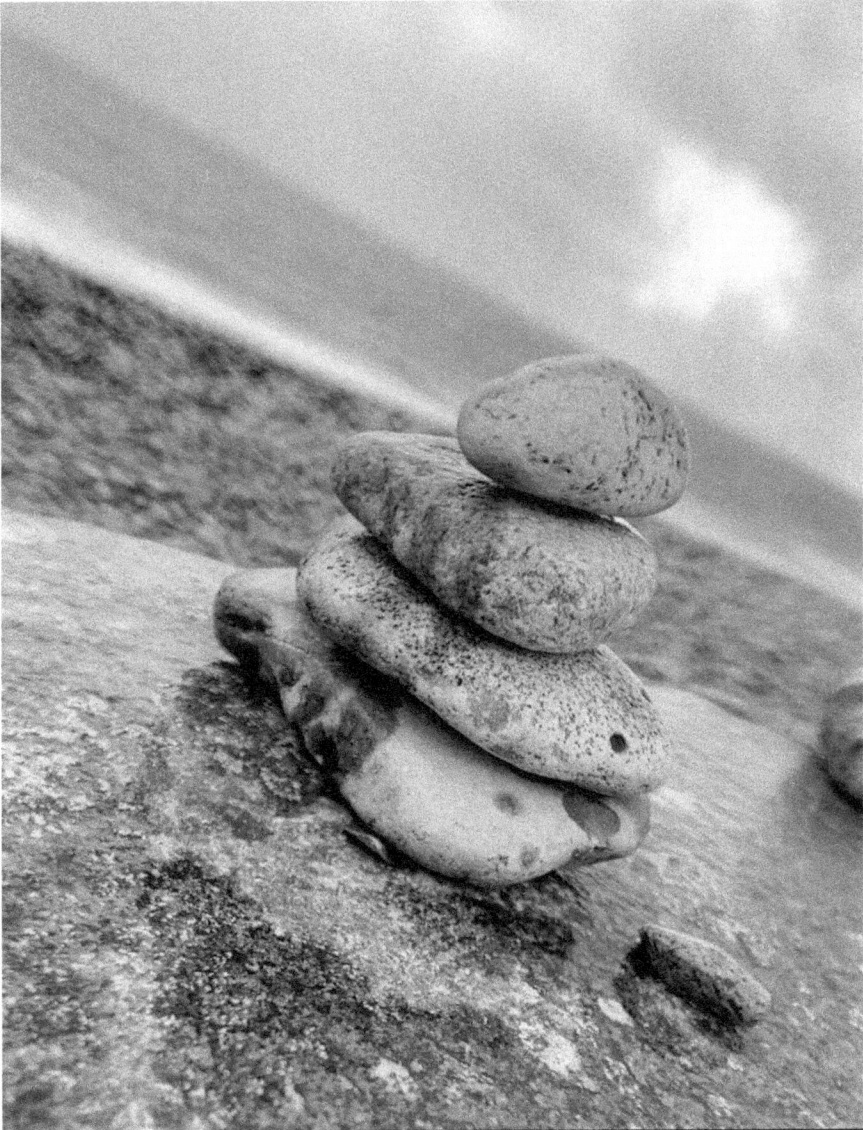

Nature is Resilience

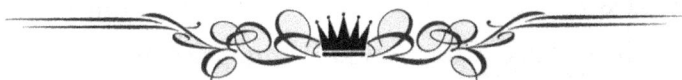

Alan Creedon

Nature Builds Resilience

When I began my healing journey, I was familiar with the word resilience. I worked in local food, helping create resilient businesses. I worked as a buyer, seller and even a grower of organic food, focused on expanding local food consumption. A resilient business was one that could stand up to market fluctuations and economic downturns, a business that could change with different trends and demands – something built to last; compact, flexible, and strong.

When I looked at my own life and state of being at that time, I realized that I was few of those things – I'm not sure I had what it took to last. I could help build a resilient business, but I was not resilient myself. I looked to others for approval and validation, I felt like a fraud and was easily offended, ready to jump to my own defense or have a go at someone else.

At one point in my life, I saw 'self-protection' as resilience. 'I can look after myself' I thought. "I don't need anyone. That's resilience."

Alan Creedon

Somewhere within me, I had lost touch with my own sense of balance. I knew I wasn't happy, but I didn't know why. I drank to hide from it, so I wouldn't have to face up to it. I was in my mid-thirties and feeling dissatisfied. I had bouts of depression and hopelessness, low moods, and very low self-esteem. There were things going on for me I wasn't aware of, I felt like I didn't have control over my own moods and my confidence was low. I was doing well in my work but in my personal life I was withdrawing. So, I decided to find out what was happening with me.

I worked outdoors at the time, I spent my time in nature, surrounded by plants. I was being shown something through watching the seasons, working with the weather, through having the wind and rain in my face and the sun on my back. I had a need for more connection, as if a quiet voice inside me was saying "this is what you need."

What followed was a wild journey of self-discovery, self-appreciation and, also of letting go, and I went to nature throughout this journey to find stability and reassurance. I began to see that I had long-held beliefs and pain from childhood trauma that I was afraid to look at. What I didn't see was what I was most afraid of actually fueled my freedom, but I had to make those first brave steps out of the situation I was in and into the unknown in order to find that path to freedom.

I let nature become my confidante, my support, my way to gain a deeper understanding of myself. And it wasn't just the natural world. It was also people. I allowed myself to become more supported by those around me, because I finally began to see that without people and their support, I was only trying to protect myself all the time. I realized that through being bullied and a very sensitive boy, I was in the habit of trying to stop myself from being hurt. I carried this habit into manhood unhealed, which meant I found it extremely difficult to trust and let my guard down.

When I started to look at myself, to connect with the truth of my experience I saw that I wasn't happy being that way. I was so involved in my thoughts all the time it was as if I missed out that there was a world around me, calling me, there for me in some way.

I got lost in the world of sowing seeds, watching plants grow, watering, planting, and harvesting. I marveled at my job, whilst seeing that all I was doing was helping to create the best conditions for the plants to grow – it was obvious that nature was doing the work of growing the food and I couldn't do it without nature.

Sometimes I would stand and stare in the market garden, taking in the scene before me, surrendering myself to the beauty of nature all around. I could see that I was looking at trees and plants, the sky, and clouds, but it felt like there was much more to it than that. I began to become aware of something deeper within nature that was calling me.

So, I listened. I listened and I followed

I found myself a year later starting a training course to become a nature connection guide because I felt that would help me deepen my connection. The training was good, partly because it involved a lot of sitting around! We would go into nature and sit. Sit amongst the trees, sit on rocks, on hillsides and near streams. The other part of the training involved connecting with senses, some guided meditations and generally preparing my body for opening- up to the world around me in a more considered and calm way.

The training helped me see that I already had a deep connection with the natural world and that I could hold space for others to explore their connection. This mainly involved helping people to relax in the natural environment using tools like Chi Gong and Yogic practices such as the body scan and through that relaxation they could open -up to the subtler energies or connections which can ordinarily remain hidden.

But What I felt Most of all was Resistance

I hated it! Hated the training (my resistance), the people who were running it were idiots (my resistance) and I could have done it so much better myself (also my resistance, all with an unhealthy dose of arrogance thrown in!). I was annoyed at what they were saying, how they were teaching it and I felt like an eejit to be subjecting myself to such nonsense. I was rebelling against 'the system', blaming others and falling into my lifelong trap of not trusting. Little did I know how the training would impact me further down the road!

They sent us out for one night to find a spot and sleep somewhere - alone, out of sight of the other course participants. I had just bought a bivvy bag and no tent. I decided to sleep in that. A bivvy bag is basically a rain cover for a sleeping bag, complete with hood and it enables a person to sleep outdoors on wet ground or even in the rain. My first outing with the bivvy bag had been a somewhat frightening experience up a hill in a gale, with the rain lashing down on me every now and again. The bivvy bag did the trick though and despite not getting much sleep that first night – I was dry in the morning.

On this particular night, it was still and a bit chilly as it was April. We were in the Lake District in the North West of England, next to lake Coniston. I sat down on the spot I chose to sleep in, and I could see for miles into the distance over rolling hills and not a person in sight, just the odd sheep going about their business. I slept fitfully. The position I chose to lie in was not comfortable and moving would have meant getting out of the sleeping bag and keeping myself warm while I dragged all my gear to a more appropriate place – in the dark!

It was a clear night, so I made the most of it, enjoying being out under the stars, moving between the feeling of discomfort and noticing the peace and beauty of the scene. I was part of in that moment. I fell in and out of sleep and, as I saw the first faint bit of greenish-blue light of early dawn appear on the horizon I fell fast asleep.

I awoke just as the first rays of sun hit my face and I noticed that there was frost on my bivvy bag and sleeping mat. I had slept out in below zero temperatures! A wave of achievement washed over me and in that moment something happened. It was the sunrise, of course, but something was happening to me, from within. I opened- up in some way in that moment. My resistance fell away and I was there in that dawn, in that perfect golden orange glow of April dawn, alone. It was truly stunning. It felt as if it had all been arranged just for me, so I could catch a glimpse of something beautiful, as if nature was saying – "look, see what happens when you really decide to slow down."

I felt calm and rested although I'm sure I had had only a couple of hours sleep. I sat up and drank in that sunrise. I was with every single millimeter of it, and I did not look away until the sun was over the horizon and too bright to observe. I felt totally energized and engaged, as if I had tapped directly into the sun's power and it had charged me up like a battery. I still had about three hours before I had to be back at base camp, so I decided to get up and try some of the practices we had been taught. I tried some Chi Gung, some meditation, tried opening the senses and bringing more awareness to sight and sound, as I had been doing anyway, without realizing it, by witnessing that sunrise and all the beauty it brought.

When the time came to leave, I felt so grounded and present I felt like I was floating. I didn't bother putting my clumsy feeling hiking boots back on and made the one-hour walk back to base camp barefoot, savouring every step as I slowly walked through bog, over stones and through streams with a big rucksack on my back. When I reached base camp, I felt like a completely different person to the guy who had left the night before, full of doubt and turmoil.

That experience sealed the deal for me, and I committed myself to spending more time alone in nature. I sat for hours, meditated, and generally worked on slowing down my body outdoors. The resistance I felt returned, but it was mainly to people and my own negative thinking but NEVER to the natural world. I had found an ally in nature – I could trust nature to never try and tell me what to do, to judge me or give me a hard time for how I felt. I met with the openness of the natural world – a place full of life, yet harmonious in some way. It seemed like the natural world was oblivious to me, just getting on with its own thing, not noticing me, sitting there with all my problems and grief.

I was beginning to open- up to the story of the life and death of my younger sister, who had severe cerebral palsy and about whom I felt deep guilt, shame, and sadness. The words were not there to describe it at the time, I just had to allow it to be, to let nature take its course with those feelings and emotions.

The more time I spent in nature the more insight I had. I started seeing answers to my problems in nature, in metaphors. If I was sad and I went to the river, leaves clinging to riverbank saplings after a flood told me 'Sometimes we hold on, sometimes we get stuck'. I was bringing meaning out of the natural world. I stayed on mountains for days on end, walked alone through forests and unfamiliar places, the more unfamiliar the better

– I knew that if I went places, I didn't know I would be more likely to entertain ideas that differed from my own long-held beliefs.

I started to see that my beliefs were like strong habits but were not who I was – like a kind of armour I was wearing. The armour protected me but also restrained me. Being with the unfamiliar helped my body and mind move in different ways, enough that I could allow different thoughts and curiosity to be present, both about my long-held beliefs and the new feelings I was having, through giving myself some space. I began to feel connected and over time, even with occasionally mind-boggling experiences, I grew to trust that nature had perspective for me – or to perhaps put it more clearly – that I had the answers I was looking for all along, but I needed that space to help trust my experience.

I went from a place of dissatisfaction in my life to beginning to feel like I was always learning. Through being open to the natural world more and more I was being more open to who I truly was and that led me to begin to heal long held grief and depression, to become ok with who I am as a person and realize that, just like the natural world, I need only be what I am and not some creation that's there to please everyone. I realized that, just as nature is, I am myself, and *that* fact would please people more. I wasn't a different person; all I was more aware. I helped my body and mind find balance through slowing and listening, allowing myself to be more open to possibility, rather than always wishing my life was different to how it was. I wasn't changed, I was liberated from my armour.

Behind every stunning piece of natural landscape there is a story. What we see is just the surface, that pleasing sight or feeling we might get from a place. But the truth is, that place only came about through massive upheaval, through the maelstrom of natural processes, which create rock, mountain, and ocean. The natural world is always in that process somewhere, from tornados to freezing cold weather, from killing heat to raging seas and back again to calm. And then there is some kind of growth, some kind of evolution. And we are part of that. Our lives reflect, in some way the turmoil, tribulations and tenacity of nature, we experience growth, brokenness, pain, suffering and challenges. We tap into joy, happiness, and love. All these 'things' are part of our nature - they make us who we are.

Through getting intimate with the natural world, I learned that I am simply an extension of it, and I can choose to work with what comes my way in the same way as a tree that loses its limb or a landscape that experiences landslide, or bushfires, or freak storms. Nature just keeps going, does not complain, remains totally connected and regenerates however it can.

We are part of that relationship and we are made up of the same stuff – at our deepest level we are the resilience from which the first life on Earth emerged and evolved. That is our history, and it is what carries me every day.

Resilience in Irish Agriculture

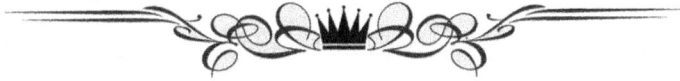

Anne Hayden

My chapter will explore resilience in an Irish agricultural context, how it affects the economic viability of farming enterprises and the psyche of farmers along with the importance of establishing a successor. This essay is written from my personal point of view as a millennial woman working in Irish agriculture and what resilience means to me. I am from the 9th generation of an Irish farming family, and I am currently undertaking my PhD in agricultural economics, and so agriculture and resilience in this profession is a topic that I am deeply passionate and fascinated by. Resilience is a term that is widely used in Irish agriculture and has two viewpoints; firstly that of family farm resilience strategies and secondly, the personal resilience of the farmer. I will discuss how it has been defined and interpreted and the unique and evolving role that it plays in Irish agriculture.

Resilience is a deeply personal and emotive concept, but it has been defined generally as the "positive adaptation, or the ability to maintain or regain mental health, despite experiencing adversity" (Herrman et al., 2011), and this trait is more common and widely experienced in my opinion among the farming community and in particular the unique role in which women in agriculture play. The decision-making process of farmers and their ability to have resilience in their chosen profession has been of a deep fascination to me, firstly watching and farming with my father and now watching my brother farm with his daughters. Their decision-making process and their ability to pick themselves up when times are tough are, from my experience, universal and captivating traits of farmers. When I think of resilience in its simplest of forms in agriculture, the words of Paul Harvey (1978) spring to mind in his speech of 'So God Made a Farmer'. Within this speech, Harvey, in a simplistic way, describes the role of a farmer and what they do from the perspective of God; he describes the requirement for farmers to be all things "I need somebody willing to sit up all night with a newborn colt. And watch it die. Then dry his eyes and say, 'Maybe next year'". These words ring as true today as they did when they were written in 1978 and are highly emotive, which were subsequently used as part of a marketing campaign by Ram Trucks in the Superbowl in 2013. It describes farmers' inherent ability to see the positive even in the worst of situations and the hope that no matter how bad a harvest, is or if an animal dies, that next year it will be better, and so they continue on. Without this inherent hope they simply would not plant the next crop or continue to farm. However, while true and beautiful, this is a very simplistic view of just one element of agriculture and resilience, and in fact, there is more complexity to the reasons why farmers choose to enter and stay in this profession.

Family farm resilience strategies are fundamentally the business decision-making process and the decisions or adaptations that farmers make during periods of great change (Macken-Walsh, 2014). These resilience strategies include joint farming and farm partnerships which formalise farmers' collaborative work (Macken-Walsh, 2014). This is an important part of resilience in Irish agriculture, and the resilience of the farmer cannot be looked at in isolation but must also include the resilience of the farm itself. Without the ability of an Irish family farm to have resilience and resilience strategies in place, it is not possible to remain technically or environmentally efficient and this in the long term, therefore, has a significant impact on the economic viability of the enterprise. There are distinct regional variances in farm sizes and type in Ireland, which contributes to the economic viability of the agricultural enterprise (Matthews, 2014). The relative economic importance of agriculture differs in each local region and in each of the main agricultural enterprises. Agricultural activities, the type of enterprises, and the level of employment in agriculture vary spatially due in part to physical and climatic factors (Donnellan et al., 2019; Matthews, 2014). When the economic viability of Irish agriculture is examined, it is found that there are significant discrepancies in farm type and profitability where the majority of agricultural sectors (bar dairy farms) have low profitability, and so a large proportion of these farms rely heavily on Common Agricultural Policy (CAP) support for income (Donnellan et al., 2019). The type of farming activity that is undertaken has a direct impact on farm viability and reliance on support-based payments to keep these farms financially viable (finish this thought). As a consequence, any policy changes to Ireland's CAP payments or to the support payments to these low profitability sectors have significant effects on family farms and there viability. This poses the question as to why young farmers would want to enter or take over these enterprises that are not economically stable.

The ability of family farms to have resilience strategies in place is also largely dependent on the personal characteristics of the farmer and whether a successor has been established. The relationship between agricultural succession and economic viability farms can thus be characterised as circular and interdependent (Duesberg et al., 2017). This relationship is also complex but can be crudely simplified thus: that the direct economic viability of certain farming types has an immediate effect on the willingness of a successor to be established; however, without investment in new technologies, these farms are likely to be less profitable, but it is more likely that only younger farmers will make these necessary investments (Calus et al., 2008). Traditional attitudes and values towards farming in Ireland still persist, and in particular, the presence of a male heir is seen as an important factor in the decision to continue the family farm. At present in Ireland, the workforce of Irish women in farming is only 12% which puts women in the minority, however, the role that women play in Irish agriculture is extremely important. As the majority of Irish farm types (bar dairy) relies heavily on CAP payments for economic viability, levels of off-farm employment are extremely high, and often it is women who take on these roles and make substantial contributions to the family home and the farms' viability as well as performing non-paid roles on the farm but yet are not considered as farmers. Young Irish farmers, despite the very volatile prices and high reliance on subsidies and the need for off-farm employment, still continue to enter and stay in farming. The reasons for this are complex but include a deep attachment to the land and the positive attitude and resilience to keep going in the hopes of making the enterprise viable, as well as a sense of duty.

The issue of succession and economic viability of these farming enterprises are intrinsically linked; however, there is a third more complex and nuanced factor of identity and sense of place, which also influences a successors willingness to be established. The concept of being attached to the farmland and how it is seen as not being solely for the production of agricultural goods but offers a wider meaning of social belonging by attaching these farmers with and within the wider community in which they operate. These experiences and the links that these farmers feel to the land and their rural communities, as well as their homeplace, determine whether successors wish to return to live and work in these rural locations in the future (Cassidy, 2010). As a result of this attachment to place and duty, land mobility in Ireland is low in an international context, and Irish agriculture is characterised by small average farm sizes with an ageing farming population (Banovic et al., 2015). This idea of place and belonging also affects the wider community is profoundly emotive and plays a central role in young farmers, both men and women, undertaking this profession, and it is their personal resilience, which helps to keep them in this role. Resilience can also be seen in older farmers with their reluctance to retire from farming completely. In studies by Duesbery et al. (2013) and Bouge (2013) found that farmers tend to continue farming not for economic reasons but for the intrinsic value and that many farmers attitudes played a vital role in this as they acknowledge that many farmers "simply would not know what to do" after they retire. This passion and resilience in farmers both young and old it seems keeps them returning to the land on which they are from and to the farming profession, which is compounded by the impact of belonging in the wider community in which it is set despite the poor economic viability.

The COVID-19 pandemic has had an irrefutable effect on society and the way we live and interact together, and without a doubt, it has had an extremely isolating effect on many Irish farmers. Many of these farms are small in scale, less economically viable and so rely heavily on off-farm employment to sustain these enterprises, which ceased due to the pandemic. As these farms are often located in geographically isolated areas, the long-term impact that this level of prolonged isolation has had on farmers away from the local community, which adds greatly to their sense of belonging and willingness to undertake this profession, will remain to be seen. However, given how strongly farmers display the necessary skills for resilience in their day to day life pre-pandemic between low incomes, price volatility, reliance on subsidies and off-farm employment for economic viability, as well as often working in isolation, farmers, in my opinion, already possess the necessary skillset to overcome these effects. It is important to recognise while perhaps these farms are not economically viable, they do provide essential services of not just food production but also conservation and protection of the rural landscape. Farmers throughout the pandemic have been key workers as they still had to continue to care for their animals and the land they farm. As I reflect on the key feature and perhaps the most important lesson that I have learnt in my 28 years as part of a farming family, it is the concept of the always present idea of hope and faith in better times. As a wise farmer once said to me, the impossible just takes a little bit longer, and this is, in my opinion, the key driving factor that helps Irish farmers to be resilient. Without hope and persistence, it simply would not be possible for these men and women to continue to work or enter into this profession, and I see this first hand in the way my family has farmed for nine generations and hopefully many more to come.

References

Banovic, M., Duesberg, S., Renwick, A., Keane, M., Bogue, P., (2015). The Field: Land mobility measures as seen through the eyes of Irish farmers 15. Calus, M., Huylenbroeck, G.V., Lierde, D.V., 2008. The Relationship between Farm Succession and Farm Assets on Belgian Farms. Sociologia Ruralis 48, 38–56. https://doi.org/10.1111/j.1467-9523.2008.00448.x

Bogue, P., (2013). Land mobility and succession in Ireland, Research report commissioned by Macra na Feírme in partnership with the Irish Farmers Association, The Agricultural Trust and the Department of Agriculture, Food and the Marine.

Cassidy, A., (2010). 'I'm not going to be able to leave': The impact of belonging to the Irish farming community on university students' life experiences and transitions to adulthood. 405.

Donnellan, T.M., Hanrahan, K.F., Lanigan, G.J., (2019). Hobson's Choice: Finding the right mix of agricultural and environmental policy for Irish agriculture [WWW Document]. AgEcon Search. https://doi.org/10.22004/ag.econ.289828

Duesberg, S., Bogue, P., Renwick, A., (2017). Retirement farming or sustainable growth – land transfer choices for farmers without a successor. Land use policy 61, 526–535. https://doi.org/10.1016/j.landusepol.2016.12.007

Herrman, H., Stewart, D.E., Diaz-Granados, N., Berger, E.L., Jackson, B., Yuen, T., (2011). What is Resilience? Can J Psychiatry 56, 258–265. https://doi.org/10.1177/070674371105600504

Macken-Walsh, D.Á., (2014). Strategies of resilience: Cooperation in Irish family farming.

Matthews, A., (2014). The agri-food sector, in Newman, C. and O'Hagan, J. eds., The Economy of Ireland, 12th edition, Dublin, Gill & Macmillan, pp. 287-311. pp. 287–311.

Self and Resilience

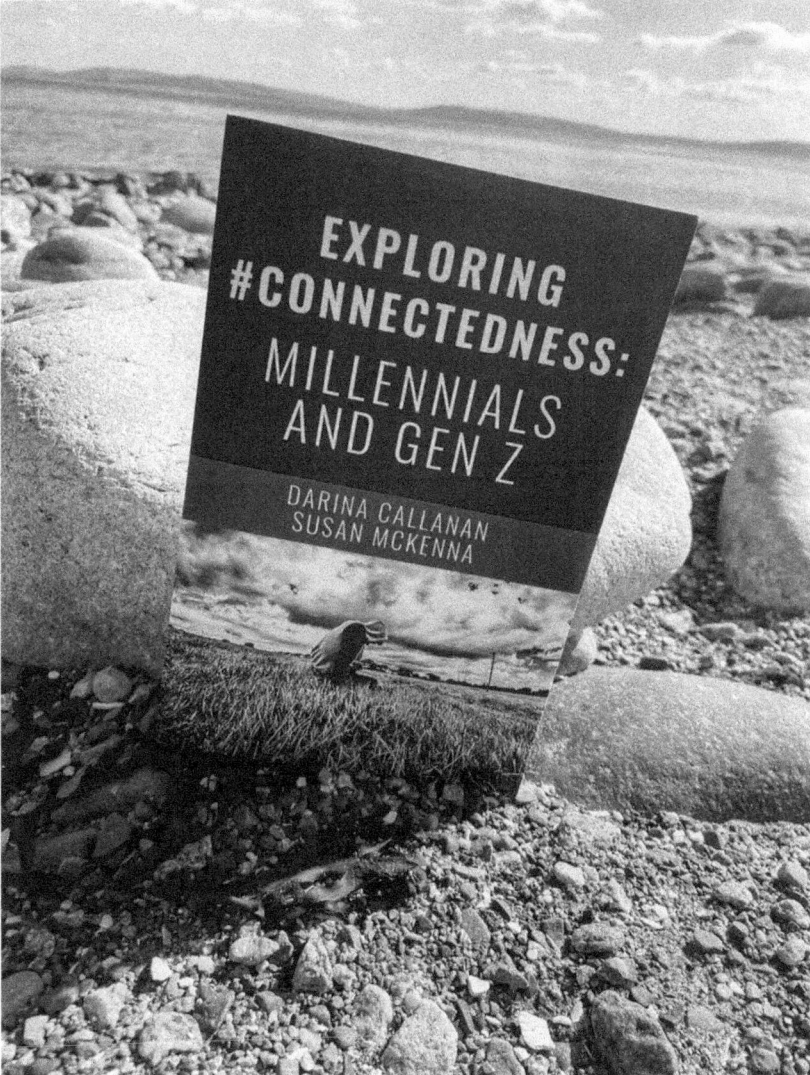

Body Image Resilience: The Millennial Crusade for Acceptance from a Culinary Perspective

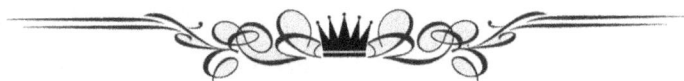

Cathy Fitzgibbon aka "The Culinary Celt"

"You are not a drop in the ocean. You are the entire ocean, in a drop"

– Rumi

The Perfect Storm

The ongoing global environmental crisis, a global pandemic and subsequent economic crisis have been of paramount importance in influencing millennials when it comes to their food choices. These external factors play both a direct and in-direct pivotal role in terms of our overall worldwide food consumption patterns. The journey of this resilient generation into adulthood, having been heavily accompanied by financial upheaval, technological transformation, and both political and social movements has been a huge learning curve requiring them to evolve and adapt in what can only be described as brave, courageous, and highly commendable ways. The culmination of this collective uncertainty has created a generation tentatively riding the cusp of a wave in terms of

71

shaping new trends and making informed choices when it comes to their image and self-esteem.

The Deloitte Global Millennial Survey (2020) recently revealed that Millennials, amongst the other younger generations, remain resilient in the face of adversity. However, on the contrary, this may not reflect the overall individual daily insecurities of these beautiful people. Unique in their ways it may be hard at times for them to find their place in this uber-connected world. They are constantly bombarded on a day-to-day basis, by a plethora of marketing techniques designed to influence their insecurities when it comes to food.

Being dubbed 'The Resilient Generation' it is heart-warming to see the determination in this generational cohort and their ongoing efforts to drive positive change in their communities and around the world globally. However, driven by this united sense of collective respect and responsibility which at times, may overshadow personal insecurities concerning their body image.

Ripple on the River: The Psychology of Eating

According to Rolin *et al.,* 2018 resilience is not only crucial in crises situations, but it's also a helpful feature in dealing with everyday life. Research studies by Izydorczyk *et al.* (2019) show an association between lower levels of resilience and stronger excessive eating patterns triggered by food appearance, smell, or effortless accessibility to food. When we are busy, preoccupied or stressed we tend to consume the quickest most comforting foods that we can find. This quite often can be in the form of fast-food takeaway convenience options rather than more nutritious fresh fruit and/or salads options. This may not be intentional when the brain is distracted, but food may often be consumed then to make us feel better. In the long term, these types of food choices do not address the underlying issue affecting our emotional mental state. It is interesting to note that a higher level of self-esteem among young people, both men and women, is an important psychological intervening variable in generating healthy eating attitudes (Izydorczyk *et al.,* 2019).

Unintentionally, millennials have grown up in a society that tends to promote and reward external beauty and physical attractiveness. Bearing this in mind, it's inevitable that a large portion of this cohort, and in particular the *vulnerable*, will feel a wave of pressure to keep up with or maintain appearances with the result that some will suffer from anxiety, depression, eating disorders, low self-esteem, and body confidence issues. When it comes to food no one size fits all and I continually championed this important truth. Having researched various diets over the last three decades and in later years discussed and learned about them in greater detail with millennials and a variety of peer groups, both face-to-face and online via my social media platforms. I find it fascinating that at times, that a large proportion of millennials don't seem to take the time to understand their bodies, by way of eating behaviours, food triggers and consumption patterns when it comes to their food purchasing decisions. They tending to be more influenced by marketing and perceived notions in terms of what's on-trend thinking these will work to make them feel more body confident. From Intuitive Eating to Keto diets, Mediterranean diets to Low-Calorie diets I've seen them all in some shape or form. This generation are now presented with more food choices than all the earlier years of my life put together! However, it's not to say that this multitude of food choices comes with additional benefits. New age food choices tend to favour the large multinational food companies whilst the undercurrent of supporting local producers is still there, bobbing away, trying to keep afloat, grounding this generation as a beacon of hope, and directing them to come safely back to shore.

Cathy Fitzgibbon

Ebb and Flow: Food Education

"Comparison is The Thief of Joy" – Theodore Roosevelt

Over three years ago I embarked on a journey creating and launching my brand *The Culinary Celt*. Deep down I wanted to be a changemaker and leave an important legacy in terms of food education, by way of imparting my unfiltered knowledge about food and how to push through the noise when it comes to the way that it's marketed.

At times food marketing can be a beast and raise its head in the form of *the Lough Ness Monster*! In the previous volume of this book series in my chapter titled "The Millennial Appetite for Culinary Wellness" I lay bare about the power of nutritional foods and how they can often be forgotten in the daily lives of this fast-paced generation, even though consistent healthy food choices can help counterbalance low mood, low resilience, and concentration levels, optimally nurturing both brain and body.

From an early age, millennials have been instilled with the notion of *'Comparative Culture'*, having grown up over decades of continual connectedness. This generational cohort is presented with the illusion of being in control when it comes to their body image. From my experience, acceptance of others seems to take centre stage. However, this may not be evident when it comes to self-acceptance and resilience on a personal level.

There is an apparent drive for perfectionism when it comes to body image and with this comes a skewed notion of 'being enough'. The millennial cohort tends to lack a sense of self in this shared community, where it seems that the sum of the greater collective can at times fuel an epidemic of anxiety, lack of self-belief and comparing judgment. As food fuels our body this unfortunately may at times be the catalyst that individuals turn to in times of low resilience and personal critique. Is it Instagram able…will I be accepted…what filter will make me look better…the list goes on and on!

Lifebuoy: Eating Healthy Boosts Resilience

As humans, we biologically adapt to our food environments. We tend to eat what is convenient and available with the least amount of energy required to obtain it. On one hand here, in what's classed as developed countries, we have a surplus of very accessible, inexpensive food which is readily available, convenient, and heavily marketed as ideal mealtime options. Whilst on the other end of the spectrum, education of nutrition and modern cultures have not kept pace with these changes in the food world. Concerns such as being overweight and worrying about food have been a result of this mismatch between human biological predispositions and the current food environment.

There are several ways that greater resilience can be built to alleviate stress. Diet is key in terms of body resilience, as eating the right foods and boosting the intake of certain nutrients can dramatically help increase energy reserves equipping us to better deal with life's challenges. When it comes to feeling resilient what we eat matters. If stressed our body may become fatigued, which in turn may lead us to eat high-energy foods options such as sugars and refined carbohydrates as a pick me up!

A bespoke integrated approach tends to work best when building resilience around food. These words of India. Arie's song beautifully reflects the uniqueness in us all when it comes to facing head-on body resilience, through what I describe as a distorted culinary lens:

"When I look in the mirror and the only one there is me
Every freckle on my face is where it's supposed to be
And I know my creator didn't make no mistakes on me
My feet, my thighs, my lips, my eyes, I'm loving what I see
I'm not the average girl from your video
And I ain't built like a supermodel
But I learned to love myself unconditionally
Because I am a queen...

Sailing Upstream: Food-Focused Mindset

Staying connected remains a way of life for millennials. The internet provides this unlimited access to information, generating a heightened awareness in relation to food tangibility that connects how we fuel our bodies via our natural environment. Good food choices are a positive and tangible way to empower facing daily body image insecurities. Food that is grown and consumed in its natural intended state helps bring about a better understanding when it comes to self-esteem and body image resilience. I have begun to call this new-age conscious state - hosting a 'Food-Focused Mindset'.

Thankfully, millennial consumers are considering foods that have been produced sustainably. A primary concern for them lies in transparency, particularly when it comes to how food products are manufactured and what's in them. However, we all play a role in terms of the health of the planet, especially when it comes to the greenhouse gas emissions caused by our food systems. So, our day-to-day food choices become extremely important in aiding the overall reduction of our carbon footprint.

Like lighthouses at sea, which for centuries have helped bring boats safely to shore, I view the multitude of social media platforms to be the new-age catalyst and enabler of educational shifts, that are empowering millennials to select and consume more wholesome, natural, and less ultra-processed foods.

Safely Ashore: The Future of Food

Innovation and technology will help us be more conscious of our ongoing food consumption patterns. Figuring out a secure, sustainable, and fair food system for our planet has become one of the most defining issues of our time. Where we go from here ultimately depends on our individual resilience and how our thoughts and perceptions of body image from a culinary perspective feed into the collective sum:

"Find the love you seek, by first finding the love within yourself.
Learn to rest in that place within you that is your true home"

– Sri Sri Ravi Shankar

References

Deloitte (2020) "Global Millennial Survey", available at https://www2.deloitte.com/global/en/pages/about-deloitte/articles/millennialsurvey.html, accessed at 17:25, 6th February.

Izydorczyk, B., Sitnik-Warchulska, K., Lizińczyk, S., & Lipiarz, A. (2019) "Psychological Predictors of Unhealthy Eating Attitudes in Young Adults", *Frontiers in Psychology*, (Vol.10), pp. 590, available at https://www.frontiersin.org/articles/10.3389/fpsyg.2019.00590/full, accessed at 14:35, 10th January.

Rolin H., Fossion P., Kotsou I., Leys C. (2018) "Considerations sur la resilience: trait ou aptitude?", *Revue Medicale de Bruxelles*, (Vol.39), pp. 22–28, available at file:///C:/Users/cfitzgibbon/Downloads/rmb-1367%20(1).pdf, accessed at 12:15, 13th March. 10.30637/2018.17-050

Diagnosis: Resilience

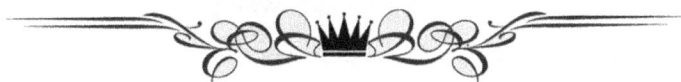

Jantien Schoenmakers

I didn't even know I was pregnant.

In the middle of that fateful Thursday night in August 2008, I woke up. My stomach was hurting so badly I was about to throw up. I went to the bathroom, sat on the toilet and realised I was bleeding. Had my period come early? I didn't think I was due one, but stress and other outside influences can affect the menstrual cycle. This didn't feel like a regular period. The cramps were so bad I had to crawl back to bed and by the time I laid down again, this nagging feeling made me go back to the bathroom. Hours went by, sitting on the toilet in the dark bathroom wondering what was going on. Things always seem scarier at night when it is dark and you are alone in pain.

Finally, daylight came. I had come home to Rotterdam to help my mother with a hospital appointment, but I had to excuse myself as I was in no state to go with her. She tucked me into bed and I finally fell asleep. When she came home two hours later, I woke up and my lower belly still felt like it was in bits and I was still bleeding. The doctor was called and he told us to come in immediately.

As we arrived, he made me do a pregnancy test as he thought I might be having a miscarriage. The test came back positive. I was in shock; I didn't even know I was pregnant? I had regular periods; I took birth control. He told me to go to the hospital and that he'd call to let them know I was on the way. As going by car would be faster than waiting for an ambulance, he suggested my mother take me and to tell the police what was going on if they pulled us over.

In the chaos, my mother had locked us out of the car. She told the doctor who came out of the building armed with a clothes hanger and got us into the car faster than you see in most movies and sent us off.

When we entered the hospital, they took my blood and realised my thrombocytes were 40, where normal values range from 150-400. If they were to do the emergency D&C right there like they wanted to, chances would be high that I would bleed to death. The ER doctor consulted with the haematologist, who put me on a high dose of prednisone to get my platelet levels back up and made an appointment to do the emergency surgery the next week.

I got sent home armed with my prednisone and painkillers and finally got a proper night's sleep.

A week later, my body had reacted well to the prednisone and my platelet levels were good enough for surgery. Fasting for 12 hours beforehand, I had asked my then boyfriend to bring me a large roll with brie when I came out of surgery. After being in the recovery room, all I could dream about was that brie. The nurse gave me some dry crackers with a slice of cheese and when I'd finished that, I told her I was still hungry but that I was looking forward to my sandwich. She told me I probably wouldn't be able to keep it down after the anesthesia had worn off. My ex walked into the room a few minutes later and they both watched in awe, seeing me eat that brie sandwich in about 2 minutes flat.

The haematologist came to see me after surgery and told me to come back a week later. Not only to check the healing progress, but also to try and figure out why my platelets were so low in the first place and to get me back off the prednisone.

The next week I found out that the haematologist I had seen, was the emergency doctor and I got another one as my consultant. She told me the other doctor had gotten me off the prednisone too fast and that's why my platelet levels kept dropping. The advice was to do a full 3 month round of prednisone to try and stabilise the levels. That would mean a full course from September until Christmas and I would slowly come off it after Christmas, but I'd still have to come in to get my blood levels checked on a regular basis.

Christmas was around the corner and I slipped into deep depression. This was amplified because of the extreme weight gain and the effect prednisone had on my mental health. The dark winter season. Seeing more of the hospital than my own home. Not knowing what was going on, why it was happening and what would happen with my blood levels if I came off it this time around. After one of the blood checks where my levels were solid, I went to the tattoo artist and got "dream" tattooed on my wrist as a permanent reminder that this would be temporary and to keep looking forward.

In February I finally got fully off the prednisone, but again my blood levels dropped. There was a clinical trial for a new medication called rituximab and the consultant told me she heard good things about it. She asked me if I wanted to be in the study and that it would be a tough one and also that I had to do a bone marrow biopsy to see if the problem with the lack of platelets could stem from problems at the source – production site. I told her I would do anything it takes because I had been educating myself these last few months on the function of platelets and their role in the body. Realising not having enough of them could quite literally kill me. The rituximab trial meant I had to go to the hospital once a week, to get a 3-4 hour IV. Having pretty much lived in the hospital during the months before, I didn't mind at all. Day one of the treatment, bone marrow biopsy was about to happen. I was told to lie down in the fetal position so they would have easier access to the hipbone from the back. From the corner of my eye, I could see the needle and by the time I felt it against my skin, my body spasmed to get away from it. On the second try my mother held my hand but as I didn't want to hurt her, I cried into my pillow instead. I could feel the vacuum from the syringe when they took out the marrow, but thankfully that was over fairly quickly.

After I calmed down, she asked to put the IV in my hand so I could move around during treatment. Normally I asked to put IVs in my elbow as I got anxious about not being able to use my hand. The first treatment went fine and my mother took me home to Amsterdam afterwards.

After a few days at home, my joints started to swell up. I thought it was just my body being stiff from being in recovery and not moving around as much as I was used to. I started to have trouble walking, with general movement and the next day, even lifting up my drink became too much. I put it on the arm of the couch, held it there so the glass wouldn't fall off and needed a straw.

I took the train from Amsterdam back to my mother in Rotterdam. As I slowly made my way down the steps, my mother got a seriously concerned look on her face. She asked what was wrong and I told her what happened with the movements. The next day we drove to the hospital for the second treatment.

They put the IV back in my hand but as I lay down in the bed an allergic reaction happened. I had a panic attack. My tongue started to swell, I got red spots all over my face, neck and chest, my blood pressure dropped. My mother called for help and as my breathing got blocked, I got intubated. I needed a blood transfusion to flush out the medication. Antihistamines to make the allergic reaction and swelling subside.

To this day I'm not sure if trauma blocked the memories, if I was unconscious at that stage or if they put me under. All I have are the flashbacks. I don't know if I want to know. Surviving all the surgeries and thinking you are going to die because of the medication that's supposed to make it all better ended up being another severe blow to my mental health.

After about 8 months of this incredible rollercoaster, I was back at square one. Not knowing why my platelets kept dropping. Not wanting to go back on prednisone knowing how my mind and body felt while taking it. Another appointment with the hematologist and another with the rheumatologist, as it was discovered I had an arthritis flare and that's why I couldn't move. My mother asks: "Could it be Lupus? It runs in the family…"

And all the pieces finally fell into place.

The resilience I got during this extremely stressful time primarily came from my mother, supportive doctors and nurses especially that did everything in their power to find out what was wrong and keep me as comfortable as they could. They were very optimistic that they eventually would find a diagnosis and that we would be able to fix it, whether it was keeping an auto-immune disease under control or curing a curable disease. My grandmother (who sadly passed away from lupus complications in 1983), my great aunt (my grandmother's sister) and my mother have lupus, so I was familiar with it. It just never clicked until my mother asked the hematologist to test me for it.

Tips and recommendations on being your own health advocate:

- Trust your gut. If your body feels off and something feels wrong, get it checked out.

- Keep a journal from the start. Describe every single inkling that something is wrong. Keep track of symptoms and write down all the questions you might have for your doctor. They will ask if you have any questions at the end and you may blank. If you have them written down, you can find the ones that haven't been answered during the consultation and address them there and then.

- Take notes during your consultation. A million pieces of highly sensitive and overwhelming information will come at you at once. It's okay to ask your doctor to slow down so you can keep up with your notes. They understand, they see it many times a day. It's okay.

- When you are going through a diagnosis journey, try to find your tribe. A lot of diseases have their own dedicated (local) charities and Facebook groups.

- If your mental health goes down during diagnosis or while taking specific medication, talk to your doctors. It's normal and they have dedicated specialist psychologists on hand for you to talk to during your journey.

- You know your body best. Trust it, nurture it and make sure it gets all the nutrients it needs, whether that means food or medication. However, you know your body best.

- Do not be afraid to talk to your doctors if your body reacts weirdly to medication, they will help you to try find a solution

Resiliency or 'Teacht aniar'

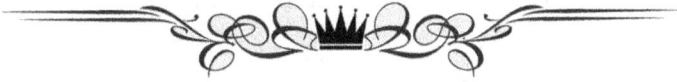

Meghann Scully

Resiliency in Gaelige (Irish) is 'Teacht aniar' which when you break it down means coming from behind. This is what I love about our native tongue, it explains words with meaning. What makes one resilient is the teachings and learnings from our past. We are not born resilient, we learn resiliency. But what exactly is it?

It means to have strength, hope in your heart and it's about being able to get back up again no matter how many times you fall. It's about healing from trauma and learning to move on with your own life by letting go of the pain. It's like playing a sport and being fit. The more often you train, the fitter you become. The fitter you are, the quicker you can recover to stay going until the final whistle.

For me, resilience came to me in the form of dealing with my parents' break up, moving around quite a lot to new towns and schools, death, dealing with breakups and managing career rejections.

Parents Break Up

My parents' marriage broke up when I was a toddler but I remember the commotion of the split. The heated conversations, the hostility in the house and the day Dad moved out. It was traumatic and unsettling as we now had to navigate through life as a new family with a new dynamic. It involved moving houses, schools and uplifting the life we were growing to know.

What I learned over the years was that not all marriages last, not all parents are meant to be together. Sometimes two people separating is the healthiest option for all involved even though it may not feel that way at that moment. Realising that my parents were better off apart was a huge moment in my own healing. My Dad was old school and strict and his mantra was "Children should be seen and not heard". My mother showered us in love and affection and never raised her voice at us. We were afraid of my father and not having him in the home house meant we could run around the house, play, shout and do as small children did without being told to stop, be quiet or be sent to our rooms.

Letting go of the loss and pain surrounding the breakup, gave me a sense of freedom in childhood but also has shown me a great lesson in how healthy, happy relationships should be. I am grateful to my parents for showing resilience and taking the very emotional step to part ways and though very painful at the time, time showed us all that we were all better off this way. My parents became friends, my Dad became very prominent in my life and we all were building a stronger and healthier family.

That time in my life gave me an education on dating and relationships and has set the standard for what I expect and know to be right in a partner, a unity and a family.

Moving

Due to my parents' separation, we had to move house. We lived in Dundrum in Dublin. It was suburban bliss. Beautiful houses with manicured lawns, numerous young families in every second house, a sense of community and safety. Shops within walking distance, the City Centre a bus ride away and great schools and sport in the area. The ideal place for a young family and a place to raise children.

All that was beginning to flourish. Marcus playing sports and in school, me swimming and going to ballet and beginning my education. I was finding my feet, my personality was developing and my memories are still fresh from those days.

Suddenly in March 1995, mid school term, we moved to Spiddal in Connemara. Not a word of Irish between us and here we were in the Gaeltacht. We rented a chalet and went to school not understanding what anyone was saying. We were the black sheep. But we had already begun to show signs of resilience. We knew to get past the breakup of our family that we had to make a new life, plant fresh seeds and water the soil. And that is what we did. We never had a defeatist attitude, we were going to survive.

The life we created in Spiddal for the next five years was one of swimming in the beach, we gained responsibility by gaining some independence. Mam would let us walk home from school, we could cycle with friends, go to the shops for sweets. It was all little acts that were part of the maturing process. We obeyed the rules and in turn were rewarded for our good behaviour.

We then moved to Ardrahan in South Galway to be closer to extended family. New school, new community, new house, a lot of change and upheaval yet again. But Spiddal was so welcoming and inviting that we were able to adapt to new surroundings and luckily these were familiar due to it being my mother's home.

How did moving make me resilient? It was all about adapting and changing. Building new connections but also keeping alive those in the previous home. It taught me that change is sometimes inevitable even when we aren't ready for it. That moving can open you to new aspects of your personality. It is a case of sink or swim and as they say in Finding Nemo "Just keep swimming".

Marcus

My big brother was the man of the house after our parents separation. He was the 'disciplinarian', the rule maker and owner of the remote control. We had that typical brother/ sister dynamic but with added father figure traits in him. I looked up to Marcus and thought he was just great. Clever, good at sports, popular and always so well dressed. He grew from a moody teenager to a gentleman.

In March 2005, we sadly lost Marcus in a car accident. Life as I knew it changed forever. The sadness, pain, loneliness, anger and depression was at times unbearable. Our home was now a dark place and the man of the house was gone.

But life had already handed me some valuable life lessons and coping mechanisms. So I did what I knew best, I adapted. I didn't want to adapt or accept this new life but I had no choice. My parents were not getting back together, we were not moving back to Spiddal or Dublin. Marcus was not returning in that door carrying his gear bag.

His death was challenging in a resilient sense. Because I was resisting grief. As the years went on, I realised being stuck emotionally in a place of loss and loneliness was only sad and lonely. That was no way to live.

Through counselling, reading, writing, sharing, talking, educating and re-educating myself, I began to take steps forward. I began to adapt. I began to heal and so the muscle of resilience began to strengthen. And little did I know, I was going to need it more than ever the following year.

Dad

The 12th of August 2006, another dark day in my life. My father, Maxie, died after a lifetime of illness. Initially, I was in disbelief. How could this happen? The flowers on Marcus' grave are still fresh and now Dad? Why me? Why is this happening? I was sixteen at the time. What could I have done that was so wrong in my short life to deserve such devastating loss?

Those thoughts grappled with my mind for some time. But again, I had to keep swimming. I had my leaving certificate ahead of me, a time of opportunity and positive change. Marcus helped me to study up until he died so I was going to use his strength to guide me through that year. I would leverage the pressure from my father to do well and gain access to University. Sometimes, I reflect on that year and realise it was that resiliency within Marcus, Dad and I that drove me on, kept me going, studying and focusing.

Now, all these years later, I realise that the two hardest lessons in my life are the reason I am the person I am today and that I will keep going, stroke after stroke and if I feel I need help, I will ask someone to throw me a buoy. Because being resilient is about bouncing back and sometimes you need someone else to assist you along the way.

Break Ups

As Sheryl Crow sang "The first cut is the deepest". And never a truer word sang. Our first experience of love is usually the worst breakup because it is the first time we felt that searing pain and loss and more often than not, we are younger. We aren't as emotionally equipped.

I went through my toughest break up when I was in the midst of my grief. I was struggling mentally and emotionally with the loss of Marcus and Dad. I was in a relationship for a number of years when the large wave of grief blew me off my feet. I could not comprehend anything anymore. I needed to be alone although I felt extremely lonely. I knew I needed to walk this path on my own. I had bottled and battled with the rising tide of grief for many years and now it was time to take it on.

That break up taught me many lessons. Grieving the loss of a relationship is similar to grieving the death of a loved one but at times feels completely worlds apart. You want to talk to your ex but they simply do not want to talk to you. You want to talk to your loved one who has died but they aren't here in person. The internal dialogue and sense of abandonment on both sides is crippling.

But you can and you will get over the break up. It takes time and also a lot of personal work. You begin to realise what you want and you need in a partner. And when you become strong mentally, when you become happy with being who you are and enjoying your own company, then you can make way for someone who can join you on your journey.

Again, it is all building a resiliency within you. You may find a new relationship and realise that it isn't right and suddenly ending something that isn't going anywhere isn't as difficult, Yes, it can hurt, that's normal but it doesn't hurt as much or for as long because you know you made the best decision for both of you in the long run.

Career

In our career we face more rejection, job losses, unanswered emails, workplace conflict, money issues and power struggle. In a relationship, it's two people navigating. In a work environment, it is numerous, sometimes hundreds or a large corporation with 1000's. There are a lot of personalities, cultures and diverse people. There's the uber confident, the timid, the bossy, the pushovers, interns, management, middle management, CEO's etc.

Work cliques form, friendships, flings, relationships. You see marriages, babies, mortgages, breakups, many life changing moments happening at all times. It's a feast for the senses.

It can be fulfilling, draining, happy, stressful, worrying, exhilarating and so much more and that can all happen in one day. If you are in any way battling mentally, work environments can feel exhausting. It's like swimming in a storm every single day. Not advisable by any means and usually all beaches are shut off to the public during a storm. So just imagine, you ignore those signs and you keep swimming. It is not going to end well.

But working in the above environments is what builds resilience. I am happy and healthy within my working world now because I have dealt with rejection, job loss, pay cuts, unpaid work, workplace mistreatment on a very high level, nasty emails, job security threats, you name it, it all happened. We spend so much of our lives working that we need to make sure we are working in a place we love. To achieve that, you must work inward. Work on yourself, your health, your wellness and turn all the negative aspects into making yourself stronger and even more resilient.

To conclude, life throws us many obstacles, challenges, highs, lows, and everything in between. We are all dealing with something daily. Much like the ocean, the sea can be choppy, cold, calm, warm, dangerous, inviting, fun, adventurous and peaceful. It is about knowing when to swim, when to walk along the sand, knowing when you need a wetsuit or if it's warm enough for swimwear, high tide, low tide and when to stay away. That is resilience.

Grief and Resilience

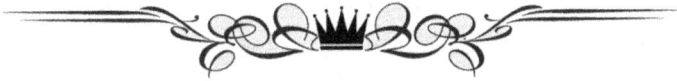

Anna Gray

I thought I knew what grief was. I thought that I understood what it does to a person, the enormous impact it has on every tiny and large part of life. I had experience of it, family members had died, I had 2 miscarriages, I even trained and worked at one time as a bereavement counsellor. I sat with people who had lost children, spouses, parents, best friends. I attended the funerals of my grandparents, friends and uncles. I know differently now. I only truly learned about grief when my mum passed away in March this year.

I thought I knew what resilience was. I'd walked through hell and back a few times in my life and always bounced back. I'd lost relationships, jobs, homes, friends and relatives. I thought resilience meant adapting well in the face of difficulty, snapping back into shape after a rough patch or being able to simply muddle on through life's hardships. What I learned very quickly (and am still learning) is that it's so much more than that.

Mum was diagnosed with incurable cancer in January, the news was a huge shock. She had been unwell, but nothing that would have given anyone cause to think it was cancer. She hated going to the doctors and as it was at the height of the covid restrictions, it was easier to avoid an in-person trip for medical care. Once her cough didn't seem to be clearing up, a private scan was booked and she had the results within 2 days. Wide spread, incurable cancer, her type called 'Small Cell Carcinoma'. It had started in her lungs, but spread around her body. Her doctor was amazed that she looked so well, considering how far gone it was, she simply felt run down and laden with a cough.

I hadn't set foot inside her house in over a year, due to the covid restrictions. I was normally there at least 5 days a week, so although we had talked in her garden, our whole family had been separated, like everyone else's, for a long time. Strangely, that part was especially hard to take, that I'd lost the last year of her life with her while she tried to stay safe from a virus, all the while she was unknowingly becoming sick with cancer. Cruelly ironic.

One of my first emotions when I found out was pure anger - anger that, in a normal year, I would have been spending that time with her, but instead we talked occasionally at the end of a garden path about what we would all do together when covid was gone. We had made plans for fancy dinners out, homely meals in, holidays and catch ups with the extended family. We said making those plans gave us something to look forward to, to get us through the tough part of the covid restrictions, it gave us something to hold on to. And then, on hearing the news, the possibility of all that was gone, taken away so very quickly and without warning. She didn't want to die, she wasn't ready. She had so much planned, things she was looking forward to doing, people she hadn't been able to see. She hadn't even had any one-on-one time with my son who was born at the beginning of lockdown, a grandchild she would never get to know properly. I'll never forget the way she hugged him the first time I brought him into her house. There was something so poignant about it, so heartbreaking.

She just looked the same to me, just like mum. She looked at me shortly after getting the news and she said – 'But I don't feel that sick and I don't look like I have cancer'. It truly was unbelievably hard to take in, almost impossible to accept as real. It still is, actually.

That initial period of time after getting the news was unlike anything I've ever felt before. The shock, the devastation, the bargaining, the anger, the utter panic, the sadness, the guilt. I felt like my world had been turned upside down, like its foundations were falling away and everything secure and comforting I had ever known was about to be ripped apart. I struggled so much with how unfair it seemed to me, she was so kind, so gentle! She had given her life to her family, devoted herself to taking care of us all, she never asked for anything in return – so surely, by rights, she didn't deserve this? Surely there was a mistake? Surely this couldn't be how life worked? How could this happen to someone with such an amazing and beautiful heart?

But of course, cancer doesn't discriminate.

Within weeks, she deteriorated quickly, her type of cancer was extremely aggressive and fast moving, spreading even further into her brain. Our immediate family were able to visit and spend as much time with her as we could, under the covid rules when someone has a terminal illness and you are helping with their daily care. We all made sure we had our time alone with her, to tell her what we felt we needed to say and to listen to what she wanted to tell us. In-between times, we had special days for her, family meals and sing-songs with our favourite old cd's and we got as many pictures of us all together as our broken hearts could cope with. In might sound strange to say, but there were magical moments, moments we laughed and cried and reminisced. Moments that were so special I really can't do them justice by putting them into words. I would catch her eye sometimes and I would see a look of such deep sadness that it crushed me all over again. She really didn't want to leave us, she really didn't have much time to prepare, neither did we.

We tried as best we could as a family to be 'resilient', to be as strong as possible for her and for each other. We pulled together, we helped each other, we all played a part in making her final days as comfortable and special as they could be. She was extremely well cared for at home, we wanted to make sure she felt how much she was loved.

When she died, about 7 weeks after her diagnoses, we were all there with her. It was 8.45pm on a Thursday night and the nurses had told us that morning that it was likely she would pass away that day. She had wanted to stay at home, she had wanted us all to be around her bed just as she was for her father years before. I thank God that she got those wishes at least, that those small comforts weren't taken away from her somehow. It's one of the only things that helps me even begin to accept what has happened. She slipped away gently and without pain. We can be grateful for that.

The nurses who came in and out of her house used to tell us we were all so resilient. That we were a strong family who, in the face of death, pulled together and helped eachother through it. I heard someone say once that being resilient is a blessing with grief because you have to find a way to carry on without them once they are gone, that you have to stay strong, you have to try to adapt. And yes, to a certain extent I believe that to be true. Losing my mum has been the biggest loss I have ever experienced, and I've had to find a strength from somewhere within me that I didn't know I had. I have children, I have to take care of them. I have to be well enough to still be their mum, to be the mum she was to me and taught me to be for my own children.

The deeper truth for me though, is that she was the most resilient of us all. We may have thought we were being strong for her, but really, it was the other way around. She faced the news of her diagnoses with grace and dignity. She wrote lists for things from explaining how to use her washing machine to how to properly clean the oven. She fought through a considerable amount of pain while the cancer progressed and her pain medication was being adjusted accordingly. She held our hands, telling us not to be sad, that we must carry on. She knew what was coming and she was still, in the midst of it all, more concerned about the impact it would have on us all than what was actually happening to her.

With each stage of decline, she could do less and less physically but yet she pushed herself. She could eat very little at times, but still showed such gratitude for the good food. She still joined in with the singing, despite knowing it would likely be the last time she would ever hear that particular song. She still did her daily crossword puzzle and beat us all at it, despite being so tired she could barely sit up for long. And, most of all, she still retained her kindness, her gentleness, her caring ways. She never once displayed any bitterness or rage, although we would never have blamed her for it. She was still her, still had that spirit we all knew and loved. She was stronger than all of us put together.

She was the one who was truly resilient. She taught me what resilience really means as she faced her own death with the courage of 100 lions. She left us all with so much to hold on to. She had been resilient her whole life, living through some difficult circumstances and tough times along the way. When I spoke at her funeral I said, 'She didn't just make us a home, she WAS our home', and it's true. She was the heart of it all and it was her resilience that kept it all together over the years.

What I'm trying to say is, no matter what losses I had before or what bereavement counselling I studied, nothing could have prepared me for losing her and for how her death shone an even brighter light on how she was the backbone of every one of us, holding us all up. She did it with and from love, no matter what came her way, she just kept going because she loved her family and wanted everyone to be happy and healthy.

Anna Gray

For me, that's true resilience - staying in a place of love within yourself when faced with such devastating news about your own health. Staying in a place of love when you don't want to die but there's nothing you can do to change it. Staying in a place of love when you aren't ready to say goodbye. For me, that's real courage and strength in abundance.

If I can learn anything from her death, it's how to be resilient like her. How to come from my heart and remain loving, regardless of the circumstances I find myself in. How to face the worst with the best attitude I can. How to keep on going, even when it feels like everything is falling apart. I miss her, every single day, and I know that will never stop. I don't want it to. But her resilience has given me a new understanding of mine.

So, I hope that people can learn from my experience. If, by sharing this story, it encourages someone to spend more time with their loved ones, to value them and to listen to what they have to say about the world, then I'm happy to share it. Part of me always assumed my mum would be there forever, I couldn't imagine it any other way. In some ways I took her for granted, over-looked her, minimized the importance of her in my adult life. I deeply regret that and wish with all my heart I could go back in time. I wish I had given her more of me, of my time and love. I used to often hear people say such things about their parents after they passed but it never really sinks in, until it's happening and it's too late.

It's very easy to get caught up in our own lives, our careers, our social life, our own problems. It's even easier to assume a parent will always be around and to act as if we will always have more time with them. To imagine that their lives are going to be threatened by an incurable illness can seem so unfathomable, as if somehow, it's something that only happens to other families. The truth is it happens and, if it does, it's so much better not to be filled with regret about things unsaid, time unspent, love unexpressed.

Reach out, if you can. Spend the time with the people you love the most, ask them to tell you the story of their lives again, ask them to teach you about the world as they see it. Learn from their mistakes and carry the lessons forward into your own life. Make memories, good ones, and savour our every single second you get with that person.

We can use modern technology for so much these days, it can be a distraction from making connections and talking to people in the room, but it can also bring us closer to people who are many miles away and help us to sustain relationships that would otherwise be distant.

For me, the meaning of resilience has changed. I used to think it was all about becoming stronger, harder, steely in the face of adversity and succeeding through sheer force of will. I now understand that to be truly resilient, we have to have compassion for our suffering and pain, we need to use it to make us softer in our strength, more loving towards our fellow human beings.

With so much in life, we will be enamoured, excited, elated and vicarious. And with loss, we will become bruised, beaten, heartbroken and, with the courage to embrace it all regardless, extremely resilient.

The Power of Self-belief

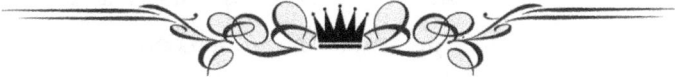

Jocelyn Cunningham

"Some people are goaded throughout life by a vision of vindictive triumph; some, swaddled in despair, dream only of peace, detachment, and freedom from pain; some dedicate their lives to success, opulence, power, truth; others search for self-transcendence and immerse themselves in a cause or another being – a loved one or a divine essence; still others find their meaning in a life of service, in self-actualization, or in creative expression".

— Irvin D Yalom

Self-belief

Self-belief plays a vital role in everyone's life, especially in the world we live in today. This can be challenging on so many levels. Life is full of expectations, disappointments, trials and tribulations. It is very easy to lose trust in situations, relationships, or environments. This can create a sense of fear around betrayal which can often lead us to rely only on our own instinct, hard work, abilities and potentials.

I feel that to reach that point of feeling, that great sense of achievement and overall balance, we should adapt a greater emphasis on self-belief. Self-belief/confidence is very empowering and can really help us in obtaining achievements, accolades, maintaining relationships, studies, in business & more importantly personal development.

Basically, what we believe will either limit or empower us.

Having good self-confidence is not something we are born with; however, we can build on this by believing in ourselves around our own personal skills, personality, presentation & behaviour. Having faith in ourselves is the first part of the battle, knowing our limits, abilities, capacities and conscious self-motivational efforts in a bid to reach our full potential, goals and dreams.

Sometimes confidence can be portrayed by our outer appearance. When, in fact, it is all about presence and behaviour. Even the most confident person has fears and triggers. Of course, but these people have become more proficient at hiding them to come across as being outwardly confident. They 'fake it until they make it!' which has become a catchphrase of millennial life.

Lack of Self-belief

It is so very easy to lack confidence after being on the receiving end of disappointment, negative feedback, or trauma. We are so good at 'doing a number' on ourselves and being reactive in our approach to various challenges and negative situations. It is incredible how we, as human beings, can allow negative narrative or experiences to undermine our confidence and overall way of being. This lack of self-belief can result in negative repercussions which may lead to feelings of upset, negative cognitive processes, uneasiness and self-doubt. Over time, a deep sense of worthlessness and inability to be our true selves in many situations can become almost debilitating as we start to lose our sense of direction and begin to neglect honoring our own personal truth. Having a negative outlook and disposition and an overall sense of not being good enough can become a way of life. Working in the capacity of a psychotherapist, I decided to raise money for a non-profit organisation that provides affordable counselling for all. I came together with two friends, and we decided on running a spinathon, whereby I would cycle on a spinning bike for several hours whilst running classes for those willing to attend and contribute. Prior to the event, I had thoughts around self-doubt. I processed them, sought supports and proceeded ahead. At the time, organising something like this was so far out of my comfort zone. The event went very well, we raised a significant amount of money, and I was overwhelmed by the support both externally and otherwise prior to, throughout and afterwards.

We can also lose the ability to be expressive regarding our opinion, thoughts, desire and feelings. It may seem so much easier to remain quiet and decide to let others determine our choices and decisions for us regardless of the outcomes. It can become both easier and habitual to remain in our own comfort zone as there is minimal risk. I took up painting over the initial lockdown and to be truthful, I had never painted prior to this. I found it both therapeutic and exhilarating and most certainly far out of my comfort zone. Below is an example of one.

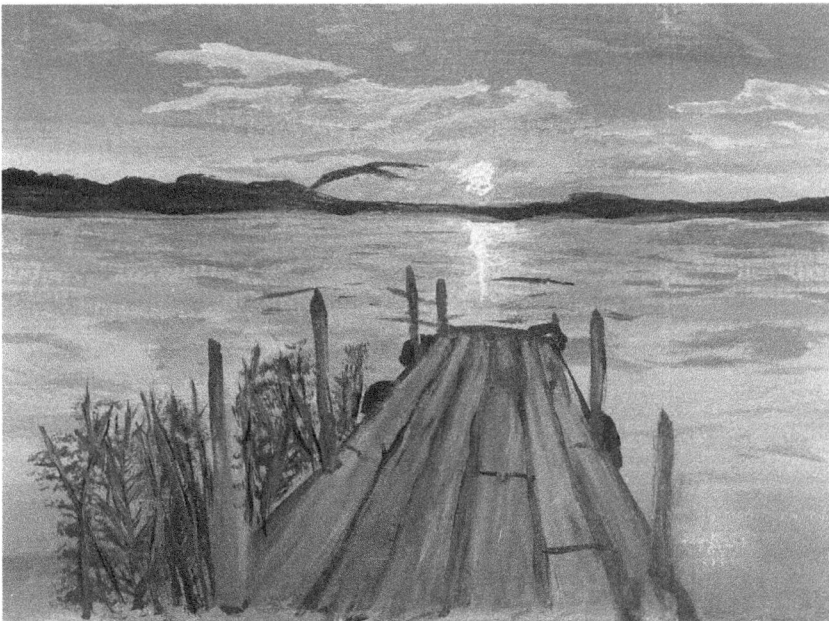

My friend named it 'Light, Peace & Hope'

The Importance of Self-belief

Having a strong sense of self-belief can make life that little bit easier on so many different levels. It would mean that facing challenges and obstacles wound not be so cumbersome. The sense of dread or debilitating fear would lessen greatly. A person would be more socially competent which would lead to handling social situations and experiences with confidence. By believing in ourselves, we trust our decisions, choices, awareness and thought processes. This inner confidence emanates through our presence, behaviour and ability to engage successfully. How we portray ourselves via appearance and presence encompasses the impressions and attitudes we have of ourselves in relation to skills, abilities, intelligences, feelings and views.

With a good sense of self-belief, we become more proactive rather than reactive, assertive rather than passive and more self-aware. Our communication skills become clear, concise and comprehendible. You are more likely to reach your goals & ambitions with a more positive outlook and attitude. It can take a lot of practice, patience and self-compassion to become more confident and it will be an ongoing journey throughout your lifetime. There is an abundance of self-help books available both online and/or on various bookshelves presently. There is also the option of seeking guidance and encouragement through a qualified therapist. I do not have to emphasize the importance of ensuring that the therapist you decide upon is fully qualified with a minimum qualification at degree level.

Negative Cognitive Processes

Human beings tend to behave in accordance with how they perceive themselves to be or appear in society. Most of us have intrusive thoughts (inner critic) which can be very damaging should we decide to believe them and let them turn into behaviours, which could result in negative outcomes.' For example, you may be considering changing job or applying for a course and the cognitive process around such a move would be a negative one, 'you're not good enough', 'you'll never follow through' which can only have a negative impact on our decision making if we were to give them credence. When in fact, we should place focus on changing them around to more positive ones. We can start this process by recognising that thoughts are in fact just thoughts. Affirming that along with other positive affirmations can be very uplifting and healing.

Making a list of the positive attributes, personality traits and capabilities may be very useful. Acknowledgment of your positives and help with our self-confidence.

Develop and Maintain a Positive Support System

Ensure that you have the right energies/people on your side. If you are feeling unsure or doubtful, sit with this feeling and decide whether it is coming from within or from someone else. If you find it too difficult to change this process, it might be in your best interest to attend a suitable qualified therapist/psychotherapist to explore the areas that are causing this inner conflict. If in doubt, talk it out. It is important that we receive the right feedback from the right sources to learn and grow. Check out how you feel with connecting with other people's energies, tune into those feelings and pay attention to them. Do these people bring out the best in you? Do you feel comfortable in their company? Do they make you question anything about yourself regarding your abilities and attributes? Steer clear of the consistent critics and lean towards the supportive people. It is true that it is not always possible but then perhaps it would be time to make relevant and necessary changes in your life to bring harmony and balance to your life.

If at first, you Fail – Try Again

It is human nature to make mistakes. It is important, though, that we do not see this a mark of failure and lose hope or give up. Instead, we should decide to learn from this and start over again. This method or approach will help us to maintain self-belief in everything we do.

Body Language

When we are met with situations that cause us to react, we reveal so much through our body language. Confidence can come across through how we hold ourselves. Starting with the right posture, having good eye contact where appropriate and a friendly face naturally reflects confidence. It is important to note that some people do not like too much eye contact and, in some cultures, maintaining eye contact is thought to be disrespectful or rude.

If you are being received as confident you will start to feel even more confident in yourself.

Discover your Strengths & Qualities

In MHFM Vol. 3 (Cunningham, 2019, p59) I noted we all have strengths, qualities and abilities which are unique to us. In fact, some of our strengths are so inherent in us that we may not even consider them strengths. Recognising such qualities, talents, gifts, natural abilities and utilising them in our everyday lives will serve us well.

In fact, research indicates that one of the best ways to boost your long-term wellbeing is to use your strengths in new ways and situations, rather than focusing on your weaknesses. For instance, a 2010 study of college students found that individuals who used their signature strengths made more progress in reaching their goals (and improving their well-being) (Linley et al, 2010) In addition, an earlier seminal study in 2004 found that certain character strengths, including hope, zest, gratitude, love, and curiosity, show a stronger link to life satisfaction (Park et al, 2004).

The use of strengths and virtues is, therefore, well in keeping with the philosophy of positive psychology; to focus on the positives in your life, not the negatives!

Do not Compare Yourself to Others

Comparing yourself to others will achieve little, it certainly will not help with developing or maintaining your self-confidence. We are all unique in our own right, so surely, we should celebrate this. It is your life, your path, your journey. Self-acceptance, love & compassion all contribute to a better way of wellbeing. When we selfcare, we enhance our overall wellbeing which helps us to maintain self-belief. Believe and achieve. Decide on your aims/goals, set a plan in place, take the necessary steps/measures, and keep going until you succeed.

Conclusion

Self-belief, like happiness, is an inside job. The onus is on you to push yourself, strive to achieve your own personal goals, ambitions, and dreams. This will, of course, involve you stepping outside of your own comfort zone. Although this can take courage, it is always helpful to consistently remind yourself of the end game, that ultimate feeling of achievement.

On a personal level, I recall taking up cycling in 2016, with the ambition of completing a lengthy cycle within 12 months. Initially, it was daunting as I felt that perhaps I might not be good enough or capable of fulfilling my ambition. However, I kept pushing myself, reminding myself of the end game. After a year of training and completion of a few events, I successfully cycled the 'Ring of Kerry' over a few hours which is approximately 179KM. The sense of achievement and satisfaction after doing so was amazing. I truly believe that we are all capable of so much more than we realise, and this is where confidence and self-belief come into play.

Here are a few motivational pointers for millennials:

- Fake it until you make it.

- Self-belief in, self-doubt out

- Use affirmations to help remind you of your capabilities

  - ➤ I post affirmations daily via my twitter handle @psyclingqueen in the hope of helping people to frame a more positive thought process or outlook should such affirmations resonate with them.

  - ➤ 'You have the inner power and wisdom to shape your day and future' JC

  - ➤ 'Only YOU can determine your value, self-respect & self-worth. Maybe, it's time to stop focusing on self-limiting beliefs & embrace your self-worth completely. You are good enough. You are worth it'. JC

- 'The quality of your thinking determines your way of being'. JC

- Establish a good selfcare routine

- Keep a journal of your journey to reflect on for future escapades.

- Avoid the critics/energy vampires and seek out enthusiastic and supportive energies.

- Aim high but being with achievable goals initially and never underestimate yourself.

- Do not compare yourself to others, we are all unique in our own right.

- Try not to overthink things, just trust yourself and put in your best efforts.

- If at first you fail, keep on trying.

- Finally, best of luck and remind yourself daily that you deserve to feel well and happy.

References

Cunningham, J (2019) MHFM Vol. 3: *Finding balance to enhance your wellbeing.* The Book Hub Publishing Group

Linley, P. A., Nielsen, K. M., Gillett, R., & Biswas-Diener, R. (2010). Using signature strengths in pursuit of goals: Effects on goal progress, need satisfaction, and well-being, and implications for coaching psychologists. *International Coaching Psychology Review, 5*(1), 6-15.

Park, N., Peterson, C., & Seligman, M. E. P. (2004). Strengths of character and well-being. *Journal of Social and Clinical Psychology, 23,* 603–619.

Yalom, I.D., 1999: p6 Momma and the meaning of life: tales of psychotherapy. Judy Piatkus ltd.,

Children, Youth and Resilience

We are mosaics -
pieces of light,
love, history,
stars -- glued
together with
magic and music
and words.

Anita Krishan

Fall Down Seven Times Stand Up Eight – Bouncing Back from When Life Takes You to Unexpected Places – My Experience

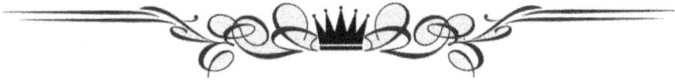

Sinéad O'Malley

Introduction

I'm a 27 year old millennial with a profound interest in psychology and mental health topics having completed a degree in Social Care several years ago. I was beyond thrilled to be presented with the opportunity to be asked to be a part of this fantastic book series. Like a lot of millennials, I've always been plagued by 'intrusive thoughts'. I regularly question myself on past decisions and I always over-analyse every minor detail of situations, coupled with always finding faults and flaws in myself. Even when I was asked to contribute to this wonderful series, the thought occurred to me – am I good enough? Could I do this? My editor assured me I could. So, here's my guest chapter. I want to commence when I was in secondary school.

School

I absolutely loved school. I can really look back at my first three years of school and say I was the most happy and content I have ever been. Unfortunately, my life took a massive downturn in my first week of Transition Year. (For people who may not be familiar with this, Transition Year is an optional year students can take after the Junior Certificate exams and prior to starting the senior cycle in your second level education in Ireland). Like many people my age, I was just starting to get comfortable in my own skin and was really looking forward to the school year ahead.

My life as I knew it changed forever on Friday September 11th 2009.

It was a beautiful, sunny day and Mam brought my friend and I to school like every other day. He was in the year below me and we had been friends since we were toddlers so I really didn't know my life without him. We had a sibling-like relationship and would laugh, joke, bicker and fight all in equal measure. We always travelled and walked into school together. Many people thought we were siblings as we even had the same surname. We walked into school that particular morning and chatted and joked as we always did. He turned to me at the door and smiling said, "Sure look, I'll see you later".

I didn't go home that evening spending the afternoon with another friend. Later that evening, I was picked up early, not knowing why. My Mam told me that my friend had taken his own life and was gone. She and I went to his home, and we were greeted by chaos. The emergency services were there, it was dark, there were red and blue lights flashing around us. The fear and wish to turn back time was overwhelming.

The following days were harrowing and I have only vague memories of them. I felt I was in some kind of bubble, floating above the nightmare. There were people everywhere, strangers hugging me and my heart was broken into a million pieces. I have a familial relationship with his parents, I have loved them all my life. I would visit them much more often, but I

114

feel I put them in mind of what he could have been, and what we would have done together, and I would move mountains not to upset them, as they have lived through every parent's nightmare already.

I didn't sleep well for a long time after his death. I also did not feel like going back to school ever again. In hindsight, I don't even know what I would have done if I hadn't gone back to school. With a lot of coaxing by my parents I eventually returned to school.

I would wake up every day with a heavy feeling in my stomach at the thoughts of having to go to school. I felt so empty and sad all the time. I had no comfort or relief and it appeared to me that everyone was getting on with their lives except me, and in my own mind, I felt embarrassed about how I was feeling. I became an expert at 'looking happy'. So deceptive – a girl who could freely walk around the school every day with a big smile when I really felt like I was suffocating and dying on the inside and no one could possibly ever understand. I believe anyone who has lived with extreme sadness can relate to the feeling of putting on a show of positive emotion for the people around you.

A Counsellor was brought into the school. At the time, I was so focused on being 'normal' there was no way I could let them disturb the wall I had surrounded myself with.

Every year, on his birthday and his anniversary, I put photographs of him on my social media accounts, not for me, but so others will remember him. I have an ongoing fear that he will be forgotten. He was such a character and would have been such an incredible adult. He made a mark on the world in more ways than one. Someone like that should never be forgotten. The vast majority of the stories we tell of him, are hilarious. We now laugh through the tears, and although he has left such a gap in our lives, his fifteen short years left so much fun and laughter to be remembered forever.

I have spent a lot of time over the last number of years through the mediums of books and podcasts in an attempt to find a quick fix for my mind. I avoided 'Darkness into Light' for many years as I feared I'd be too upset to part-take in such an emotional event. Darkness into Light is an event held in Ireland every year in communities across Ireland aiming to raise vital funds that provide free help and support for people experiencing suicidal ideation. It's an incredibly invaluable resource for people who find themselves in very difficult times. It's a fantastic event that brings huge communities together where they all meet prior to sunrise and walk together. Having completed it the past couple of years now I can honestly say it has been a form of therapy for me.

Upon reflection of writing this chapter, I am very much aware of how hazy my memories are of that time in my life. I genuinely just existed rather than embraced life. I found myself doing absolutely anything at all to avoid being on my own with my thoughts. Genuinely, if someone organised the opening of an envelope I would be there. I would do absolutely anything at all just so I wouldn't have to be alone with my thoughts.

College – Round One

After the hardship of the final three years in school, I decided to study for a Social Care degree as I felt it would be the best avenue I could take at that time. For a module in my degree, we were tasked with creating a therapeutic tool that could be used to help someone who was facing difficulties in life. I chose to write a children's story book that encompassed Elisabeth Kübler-Ross's five stages of grief model. During that time, I often wondered what stage I was at myself with my grief. I felt really good about myself after completing this assessment because I believed I could really relate to the task at hand and the core message the lecturer was trying to deliver.

Postgrad in a Pandemic

After many years of feeling huge waves of persistent, extreme sadness and feeling like I wasn't where I was meant to be, I decided to push myself and applied to go back to college. I believed it was now or never to pull myself out of the hole I was in. And I felt I was more confident at the age I am now in knowing what I wanted to do 'when I grow up'. I wholeheartedly believed there was no time like a global pandemic! I spent weeks researching courses in the Business, Marketing and Human Resource Management field and decided to apply to NUI Galway. Within less than 24 hours of my application being sent, I was accepted. This decision was the start of the best thing I could have done with my time during the many lockdowns and heavy restrictions we faced in Ireland. Being a goal driven person, I knew this postgrad would give me something to aim for and really focus on during a very uncertain time in the world. I threw myself into work with the hopes of eventually making it into campus at some stage during the semester. Unfortunately, we never did make it to campus and I, many other thousands of students, completed an entire postgrad from my bedroom at home. I can honestly say hand on heart completing the postgrad was one of the best decisions I have ever made. Not only have I learned so much in a completely different field of study, I learned so much about myself. I have gained more confidence in my own abilities and am safe in the knowledge that I can do things solely on my own. I believe my postgrad experience outranked my undergrad experience because I was still letting sadness dominate my life during the course of my undergrad whereas now I try to put things in place for myself and know the signs of when I just need to take a break and reflect on my feelings.

Conclusion

It has taken a great many years for me to actually start moving forward with my life. I won't lie or insult anyone by saying I am by no means a fully healed person. In my experience, trauma brings about so many changes in you that you develop into a completely new person and can never really go back to being the same person you once were.

I am of the strong belief that the key to being a successful, resilient human being is checking in with yourself and reminding yourself why it is that you have chosen to move forward with your life. Upon reflection of my own experience, I can say I (after a very long time) picked myself up and started healing my own wounds. I am also aware that some of these wounds will never fully heal and have come to accept that.

I admire how grief is spoken about so much now. I hope for anyone reading this that has experienced similar circumstances to mine that they can believe that life can get better. I continue to work on myself but I now do not live a life where I am completely controlled by my negative thoughts, habits and behaviours.

Learning Nuggets:

- Life can change in a split second. It's very hard trying to live in the present moment but it really is the most important way of living life.

- Try not to let external circumstances dominate your life. Bad things happen to people every day and while you can spend your time sitting around thinking 'why me?' or you can get back on track and stop wishing to change the past. It doesn't work and just wastes more of your precious, valuable time.

- Celebrate the small things. Those little wins you accomplish on a day-to-day basis can bring about more confident and positive behaviour more than you may realise. Reflect back on these wins often and be proud of how far you've come.

- Accepting who you are as a person is difficult but by doing so, you start to have faith in yourself and you can only succeed. Accept that you are not a perfect person – and no one else is either.

Let's Never Forget Our Marginalised Children: 'At Risk' and Resilience Explored

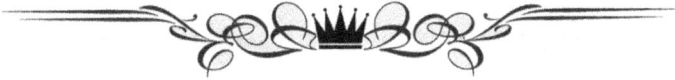

Susan McKenna

Introduction

A debate is raging in the Republic of Ireland in relation to the issue of intervention, treatment and rehabilitation of juvenile offenders. This chapter looks back to my time as a social care worker and addresses one of the intervention strategies made available by the Department of Education in the Republic of Ireland, that of the Youth Encounter Project System (YEP) and, specifically, Saint Augustine's school in Limerick city where I did a placement and then worked for a while. In fact, I worked in the centre for a period of 18 months and engaged in an ethnographic study.

By working with and participating in the wider lives of the pupils there, I came to understand the motivation behind what is largely perceived within 'mainstream' society, at least, as dysfunctional behaviour. The children in Saint Augustine's were categorised as 'at risk' by the Department of Education and I am of the opinion that once the children enrolled in Saint Augustine's School, they became less statistically likely to either remain or become involved in criminal behaviour because they had sustained empathetic education.

'At Risk' in Context

Since 1973, families with children replaced pensioners as the group most vulnerable to poverty in Ireland. While this is in keeping with other developed countries, the trend is very pronounced here. The risk of poverty with families with children is also positively related to family size and is particularly strong for families with one or more children. Irish children face higher risks of being poor then Irish adults which is a shocking fact in 2021.

It still irks me that academics argue about how poverty should be *measured*. They're concerned about the correct position of the line which measures poverty but this is of little comfort to a whole subculture of families the length and breadth of Ireland and, in particular, in Limerick city – 'my hometown' as Springsteen sings of his own hometown.

There is an association between lower social class and inferior outcomes to a whole series of measures such as infant mortality, general health, educational attainment, and employment prospects. Of course, one of the issues in post-modern life and particularly in Ireland is that we have seen massive, telescoped change in the very definition of 'family' over the past few decades. We are all aware of the saying 'give me the child at seven and I will give you the adult'. There is some encouraging evidence of the resilience of children in the face of adversity and of their capacity to make up lost ground if circumstances change in their favour and this is something my colleague Dr. Niall MacGiolla Bhuí has written extensively about. The idea of child experiences shape the adult is widely held among professionals working with children and youth even if its profound implications are not yet reflected right across Irish society's social and political priorities. And I can attest to this after two decades experience in direct social care practice and management prior to my transition to a life in publishing.

The notion that children acquire many of their characteristics from learning experiences within the family has truism status in modern thought. So does the idea that problem families produce problem children. I remember well back in my time working with disadvantaged children, a comment by my colleague Michael O'Connor who was, at the time, Director of Oberstown Boys Centre in Dublin, "If we really want to do something about tackling the roots of crime in our society we need to empower vulnerable parents working with them from the very onset when children are still at the toddler stage"

The Roles of Parents and Carers

In most societies, parents carry the fundamental responsibility for the welfare of their children. When children are in trouble it is normally the parents that are subject to blame. Parents are associated with playing a decisive role in the care and welfare of the children but there are many obstacles that may hinder or stop them from carrying out their parental functions effectively. Parents roles are often undervalued and they have to be breadwinners, housekeepers, informers of sex education, financial controllers, nurses, doctors, enforcers of the family's code of behaviour and of sanctions for breaches. They have to be shoppers, career advisors, sources of encouragement…The list is endless.

When parents fail to live up to society's and indeed to their own expectations, it is often due to adverse circumstances rather than parental indifference per se. Parents may lack the supports, the good health, the physical and the mental energy, the know-how or the emotional strength to sustain their energy over the long haul. Parents who are rearing children alone, suffer from chronic physical illness or disability, parents suffering from alcohol or drug addictions, parents with psychiatric disorders, parents with marital difficulties, parents on low income, or inadequate housing all affect their functioning as 'good enough' parents.

It is my experience that many parents are still suffering from the lack of love and security that was not present in their own childhoods. Many are also suffering from unresolved traumas. Indeed, psychology and psychotherapy note that people can only give what they themselves have already received. Given the critical role played by parents in Irish society and the challenges in the quickly changing attitudes to parental and other forms of authority in society, it seems important to note that some parents are almost certainly going to get into difficulty and, often, and it is not their fault. I have also found in my professional work that it is more productive rather than looking for someone to blame to offer parents and families active, real and meaningful supports so that they and their children will not suffer difficulties.

At Risk Status

So what doors 'at risk' status actually mean? What does it confer on a family what does it confer on an individual? To say that the family is 'at risk' is not to say that it is necessarily in trouble but rather to indicate statistically there is a significant possibility of problems. Maya Pringle back in 1974 described at risk as "being vulnerable because of the presence of specific potentially detrimental personal family or social circumstances". Her colleague Nicola Madge later described at risk as meaning to have "an above average chance of family difficulties". We can say that the expression or the term 'at risk' is not a definite term. Not all families or children who are deemed by authorities to be 'at risk' are actually in need of specific special or therapeutic interventions. Certain indicators serve as general potential factors for helping to assess if a family is experiencing difficulties.

Nicola Madge very usefully described five factors as being important guidelines to indicate if a family may be suffering difficulties. These include the age and maturity of parents, the burdens that are present and carried, family consistency and change in the lives of children, dynamics and supports within the family and experiences and characteristics of individual family members.

At a seminar held in Mary Immaculate College in Limerick city by the Department of education my colleague, Dr Niall MacGiolla Bhuí, distributed a questionnaire asking for comments by teachers of special education on what they believe to constitute 'at risk' status for children and the answers were Illuminating. I include a sample answer from one of the delegates present on that day.

"Attitude, lack of home support, lack of basic social skills, poor self-esteem, physical factors such as hunger and lack of clothing, multi problems, anti-education, emotional disturbance, poor attendance at school, home environment, instability, inappropriate parental expectations, lack of ambition, lone parents, peer pressure and learning disability."

Resiliency

Resiliency speaks to 'bounce backability'. We can think of it as emotional elasticity. The children and youth who attended the Limerick Youth Encounter Project demonstrated enormous resiliency by simply getting out of bed, often with no breakfast or parent(s) to monitor them, by walking or getting a bus to the project and for engaging in the project. Simply being there for several hours a day took them off the streets, away from potential criminal involvement and away from their more wayward peers. I am blessed to have worked with the project as it has given me a lens on life that I would otherwise never have had. One can think one 'knows' one own's city, but there are so many aspects that lie largely hidden away from sight unless one is fully prepared to embark on a journey of discovery.

Summary

The 21st century has seen many changes in the structure of societal patterns, in technology and information transmission and in cultural and religious practices and Ireland is no exception in this. Indeed, our country may well have become fundamentally unrecognisable in many aspects of our cultural norms to anyone who had left this island for any period of time and returned home to us. Children and youth deserve an opportunity to lift themselves out of circumstances that may drag them down. In this the Youth Encounter Projects blazed a trail because they embraced and engaged a resiliency perspective even before it became fashionable in working with families 'at risk'. Limerick city owes St. Augustine's Special School a debt of gratitude.

*A special mention of a wonderful human being, the ex-director of St. Augustine's – John Hanna.

References

Madge, N. with others (2000) *9 to 13: The Forgotten Years?* London: NCB.

Madge, N. (1997) *Abuse and Survival: A Fact File.* London: Prince's Trust - Action.

Madge, N. (1994) Children and Residential Care in Europe. London: NCB.

Madge, N. et al (1993) *The National Childhood Encephalopathy Study: A 10-year follow-up.* Supplement to Developmental Medicine and Child Neurology, July.

Madge, N. (Ed) (1983) *Families At Risk.* London: Heinemann.

MacGiolla Bhuí, N. (1997). *Children At Risk.* New York. Haworth Press.

Pringle, M. (1986). *The Needs of Children.* Taylor and Francis.

The Kids are Gonna be Alright

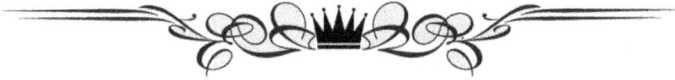

John Madden

It all happens so fast.

I lay in bed, almost afraid to move. There were a million reasons to get up, but one important one that I was terrified of kept me frozen. I lay there with that cloud of reactionary depression and anxiety like a stranglehold pinning me down. I'd been here before, I had been party to breaking such news but the old adage "the shoemaker's son is the last to be shod", however, the 'here' was significantly different this time. Uselessly, I stared at the ceiling as I hear his laughter outside amongst the other children. He does not know yet. The knot in my stomach twists and contorts even more than earlier. I do not want to see him have to go through this, it changes everything. Once he knows, his life will never be the same. He is 6.

Darren's dad died the previous night; it all happened so quickly. Upon the news breaking, Darren needed to be collected from his nannies. It was around 11.30pm and when collected he was confused, disoriented and still sleepy. "Something is going on, I don't know what, everybody is sad". Why do you say to that? "I'm not sure, buddy, let's just get you home and into your own bed, mammy is on her way back too".

"Dar, will you come in here for a few minutes, mammy and me need to talk to you?" My neighbour says, she has lived-experience of such tragedy herself. It is out of my hands, and in a few minutes, his life will change, maybe irreparably so.

He knows.

Expected reactions and startling statements

The following days were indistinguishable, brightness and darkness were the only things that discerned the differences as the days changed. Happiness was fleeting, sadness waiting in the wings for the "right" moment, never far away akin to the Sword of Damocles being held aloft by frayed and weakened threads. One wrong word, emotion, thought and it would slice through the small semblances of normality we were desperately trying to cling to. But pressure mounts and the inevitable collapses happen. It can only be likened to trying to toss buckets of water out of the Titanic. It might buy some time but you're sinking; there's no escaping that reality.

The first statement came that day; "I'm ok, I'm over it". Odd to hear, but not unexpected. The associations with the gravity of the situation had not hit home. He had not yet seen his dad's body laid out as is the tradition in Ireland. It was almost a detached response to the reality, maybe a coping mechanism to negate the plethora of emotions that were rampant in his head, and our own. Perhaps, a manifestation of denial.

The next one was terrifying, but again, not overly unexpected; "if I die, I can see daddy again". We read and hear about this quite a bit. Kubler Ross, in her writings, identifies several stages of the grieving process. None of which are linear or follow a predetermined path; but they are common to many enduring losses, but to hear it from a loved one, especially one so small in stature and low in life-experience is extremely unnerving. This would be bargaining, in the sense that we would do anything to see things back the way they were and that is not attainable.

The next one of note was different; once the funeral was over and we journeyed beyond those initial days of incessant tribulations and knotted stomachs, appetites returned but the desire to cook wasn't exactly overwhelming. That's natural enough, the culmination of stress, fear, anxiety, sadness just ties the tummy in knots; sadness and adrenaline can only sustain a person for so long and it does not nourish the body or mind. A takeaway was in order; greasy, satisfying, immediate-gratification burgers and chips, and not forgetting a sloppy milkshake... Manna from heaven, devoured to the point of absolute guilt and discomfort afterward, then came the statement, "Can we eat better food from now on, I don't want to die like daddy", a mild irony that it was uttered after the food had been consumed but still, a far cry from wanting to die so as to undo what had happened a week before hand.

A comforting network for a very brave boy

Everybody had Dar at the centre of their concerns and thoughts and that became deeply apparent as the days and weeks progressed. That was and continues to be, welcome and concerting but the resilience he unknowingly demonstrated has been an inspiration, one that we can all learn and grow from. Although he had a frontline defence comprised of amazing neighbours and individuals ready to comfort, help and whatever else was needed, he traversed much of this by himself. A defining moment of bravery happened early on; his dad's body was in his mother's house. He was told that he was under no pressure to see his dad laid out and that nobody would make him do anything that he was uncomfortable doing or simply did not want to do, but he mustered up his own courage, of his own accord and walked slowly into the room to spend time with his father. It is difficult to fathom what must have been going through his head right there and then, but he did it, at 6 years old.

The Kids are Gonna be Alright

The title of this series holds at its forefront, Millennials. Dar is far too young to be categorized as such, he's Gen Z but it is certainly the case that he has been raised by Millennials. If the children that our generation are raising have even a fraction of that kind of resilience, then we have quite a lot of hope and a good future to look forward to. We teach children a lot, but we can and should learn a great deal more from them. The light might be a little dimmer, but the flame is beginning to dance again, little by little. The memories remain, there is still pain and sadness, that will not leave but we can live with it. That, to me is what resilience is about. We learn to live with the slings and arrows of life. We learn that at times, it is unfair and other times it is downright cruel, it is how we adapt and overcome is what defines us. Owning it, engaging in open and direct conversation around it helps too. If I had a euro for every time that he has told somebody that his dad is no longer with us, I would be a wealthy man but what care we for riches when he enriches our lives daily. He owns the situation; it is his and he will discuss it with whomever he wishes to hear it. He isn't bundling up feelings or emotions and hiding them away, the story is on his terms and although it can be hard to hear somebody so young say that aloud, it is impactful. It is his way of taking ownership of the tragedy, a skill that underutilized, or maybe even forgotten by adults.

What Hurts us can Strengthen us

We are delicate, like porcelain plates at times, the fragility of life. We endure cracks and chips throughout life, fairness does not enter the equation, it's shit but that is life. We can't live in the box, encased in the safety of bubble wrap; that's not living. The cracks and chips of life change us and shape us into the people we become. The chips and cracks are manageable, granted we are never going to be pristine again, but we can deal with it. But this story isn't about chips or cracks, it's more so about when the plate shatters into something that looks irredeemable, unsalvageable, ruined entirely. We long to return to what life was like before the porcelain smashed but that's not possible. Instead, we need to work on how we can try to rebuild but in doing so, is it ever going to be the same? Probably not. We strive for 'the same' but we can do better, and maybe that is a problem for resilience in many. There is too much emphasis on 'getting things back to the way they were'. We know we can't do this, yet we bog ourselves down in trying to achieve the impossible.

There's a lesson to be learned in all of this; Dr Julie Smith (2021) provides an amazing comparison in this regard as she states, instead of looking to do the impossible, maybe we can look for inspiration in Japanese culture. The concept being alluded to is Kintsugi, it is the practice of repairing the broken object and turning them into something even more beautiful. The object is repaired, not to hide the cracks but to accentuate them with gold and celebrate their value so they become part of the story rather than the end of the story. The repair, just like recovery and healing, takes a lot of time, effort, progress, regression and a multitude of impediments along the journey. Instead of throwing what is perceivably damaged away or pretending that whatever happened, didn't happen, we give the cracks meaning and purpose by using them to enhance the things as a whole and celebrating the fact that they were instrumental in making you the person you are today. Parting words

Grief and tragedy will enter your life, you can try escape it or hide from it but it will catch up with you. How you face it is up to you. Perhaps you can draw some strength from the 6 year old's story. His is really only beginning. The trauma is the gold, his life the plate, but with love, support, and Kintsugi, he can face anything, and when there's times that I can't, I will remember this, vividly, and draw strength from it too.

'It Will Always Be Christmas in my House'

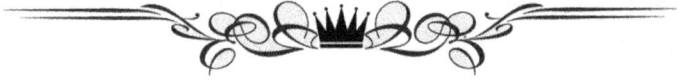

Karen Gallen

Introduction

My name is Karen Gallen and I am a mother to two beautiful teenagers, one boy and one girl. My contribution to this book is around life with my daughter who has additional needs. As this term is used quite freely for a range of needs, I will explain that my daughter has both additional physical and intellectual needs. She requires a lot of care above and beyond a peer child of her age and has been diagnosed with severe scoliosis in the lumbar spine, epilepsy, global developmental delay and a clinical diagnosis of a severe to moderate learning disability.

She is a thirteen-year-old with the average intellectual ability of a 3-4 year old. Physically, she is a fulltime wheelchair user who needs full assistance with all daily activities i.e. she needs to be dressed, showered administered multiple medications, lifted in and out of bed, have her food prepared for her to mention just some of the additional requirements.

Socially, she is like a butterfly and loves social settings and has an infectious smile and laugh that masks a lifetime of hospital, appointments and surgeries. Indeed, at this point, she has endured in excess of 30 surgeries on her back.

In my experience, a lot of parents say that they would do anything for their child, but in my case I *have* to do everything for her.

Normalising the Conversation around Additional Needs

I would hope that my contribution will normalise talking about additional needs and the impact it can have on the extended family, especially siblings. My children are very close but some days I want to be able to open the car door and 'shoo' both of them out of the car and see them run to their friends in the schoolyard. Unfortunately, I know that my daughter will never be able to do that.

I have additional responsibilities and worries around her development and medical conditions but I have also the relief of not worrying about other issues parents might have such as teen discos and late night parties. Life is about balance and I have decided to look at the positives in a situation I cannot change. There will always be childlike innocence in my home/life and Christmas and Santa will always be the best time of year in my house.

Those Conversations

I am sure most people who have children can relate to the conversation that occurs when you meet other parents. It goes something like this: "How many children do you have? Boys or girls? What do they do or what sport are they into?" A seemingly innocent topic of conversation, that is, until you can't answer some of the questions without feeling the need to explain your child has additional needs. And, then, the conversation changes and will be met with one of two responses:

1. As though you have just announced a death in the family which results in the other person tilting their head to the side and saying "That must be so hard on you" and "You were given a child with additional needs, because you would be able to cope." I wonder who makes that decision? Is there somebody in the maternity ward vetting would-be parents to ascertain if they can "cope" with a child with additional needs?

2. The overcompensating conversation whereby you are flooded with stories that start with "I know someone who has a child like yours…." Or, "if I was you, I'd get a second opinion because they might grow out of it."

Having a child (with or without additional needs) changes your life forever and unconditional love and responsibility are instantaneously introduced to your world. Along with that comes organised chaos and forever being alert for any potential dangers to which your child may be exposed to. Over the years, many people have said to me, that having a child with additional needs must make life seem out of control. But, in fact, one of the biggest responsibilities and realisations for me as such a parent is the amount of control I have. My child has additional physical and psychological needs therefore I 'control' (and I don't like the terminology) when she gets out of bed, goes to bed, gets dressed, when she eats, what she eats, where she goes etc. It can be overwhelming because if I have an off day or if I am sick, I still, somehow, need to be in control.

Consent is also another word that is prevalent in my life. Will you sign the consent form for your child's surgery? Will you sign the consent form for anaesthetics? Will you sign the consent form for Special Needs Assistant hours allocation for the classroom setting? Will you sign the consent form to share a report between different therapists? And with that, comes the fear that if I sign something that results in a negative outcome, then I am forever to blame. Heavy wears the crown.

Karen Gallen

Reactionary or Revolutionary

The above have been applicable to me since the first indication in 2008, that my child was not meeting developmental milestones at her regular developmental checks. Initially I reacted, which I think is what most parents would do. I cried and tried to 'explain away' her delays etc. by saying she was born 2.5 weeks early and asking the medical team to give allowances for her 'early birth'. I also said she was small and would catch up with babies of her age. I started to avoid meeting other babies born close to her birth date. I almost crashed into an elderly couple in the grounds of the hospital following an appointment – this was due to crying uncontrollably after yet another appointment in Paediatrics whereby there was a lot of shaking heads in sympathy by the Paediatric Consultant and Physiotherapist and a list of therapists /consultants mentioned to which she would be referred to such as neurology, orthopaedics, paediatric physiotherapist for a start.

Finally, after a few days and nights of almost constant crying, when she was almost a year old, I 'gave up' being upset. I made a conscious decision I would embrace a resiliency perspective. Realistically, I wanted to cease crying as it was not achieving anything, with the exception of making me feel physically sick and ruining my mascara. What I did do or attempt to do was to try to remain calm and take on the challenges that I could see were before my daughter rather than challenging the medical opinions I was receiving. I took every piece of information I could gleam from the medical teams and read all available information about what they were trying to diagnose. I could recite every word said to me at each appointment, along with an exact recital of how her test results were explained, to the point that at a meeting with the geneticist in Temple Street Children's Hospital she asked me what branch of medicine I was working in. Never underestimate the drive in you to protect and mind your child/the child you are caring for.

It took a while to realise that life as I had imagined it might be, had dramatically changed so I tried to be logical and do what was required such as attending every appointment offered to her. I even asked for additional referrals to Ophthalmology and Audiology to ensure that all bases were covered. I continued to plod along for approximately two years until it came to a time for her to attend preschool. This is when the revolutionary in me kicked in.

It was suggested to me by her Community Nurse who visited her at home two days per week, that I complete an application form to send my daughter to a specialised school with nurses on site. But by completing this form, it was an acceptance by me of her limitations. I was informed there were six places available and normally a low level of applications received as parents were often anxious to let their child be under the care of another outside the home/immediate family. A few weeks later, a letter arrived stating that her application was unsuccessful. I was annoyed after the effort and emotion I had put into the process. so I decided to query why she was not accepted. Basically, places were offered to children who had little physical and emotional support at home, so effectively because she had a 'good' and supportive home environment, she was refused entry.

Several other children were left in a similar position, so I decided to take action and wrote a lengthy e-mail to the mangers of the service with proposals for expanding the classroom size and relocating staff. Fortunately, they read the e-mail and met with me to discuss it. The outcome being that she was offered a place in the classroom from 9am to 2pm Monday to Friday along with two other children and the remaining children who were not offered a classroom place were given supervised play time for a short period of time each day. From that day onwards, I decided to take action rather than have a reaction (wherever and whenever possible). This, to me, is resiliency.

As a mother, father, guardian, your focus is wanting the best for your child, whatever that may be. From the day my daughter was born, I knew that my focus was going to be getting her access to the best healthcare. A mother's instinct that all was not well proved to be right. It took me three months to persuade my GP to refer her to the hospital and from three months to one year it was a constant series of appointments and approximately 25 physiotherapy sessions in Galway over a period of six months until the dreaded announcement was made that she would have her care transferred to Temple Street Children's Hospital in Dublin. It seemed like the end of the world at the time as it would mean any appointment would have to factor in a lengthy car journey, however, it turned out to be the best decision for her medically. This was a hospital specialising in the care of children and with some of the top consultants in Europe. Twelve years later and she still attends the hospital regularly.

Thirtyplus orthopaedic surgeries later and I feel like we have become friends with the Professor there. There have many little 'blips' along the way and the Professor is so calm and confident that he says 'everything is fixable'. I have to admire his confidence but after all you do want a calm, confident surgeon. Fixable means another trip to theatre – if there were loyalty points to be collected, we would be top of his loyal customer list!!!

I learned that you should trust your own instincts. As a parent/guardian, you are the advocate for your young child, so, if you feel that they are not meeting their milestones, be that from experience of older siblings or from observing other children of a same age, you should trust your instincts. Then seek the expertise of a medical professional or whatever professional help is required. Do not always accept what you are told by anyone, be it layperson or professional. Seek additional knowledge, to ensure that the medical or health professional is confident in their diagnosis or suggested treatment plan. It is not disrespectful to disagree, rather it is healthy to have an open discussion about the positive outcomes and potential negative outcomes of a plan/procedure. Every surgery requires a consent form to be signed by me, followed by an explanation of the procedure and a reminder that I am signing for 'plus additional procedures' if required when she is in theatre. As her current surgeries are adjacent to the spine (but not directly on it), it is explained that there is still a possibility of damage to the spine. This is followed by a discussion with the anaesthetics team who explain the risks of anaesthesia and that she is difficult to intubate etc. All of her surgeries to date have been performed by the Orthopaedic Team at Temple Street Children's Hospital, however I have been advised that if she ever requires any non-orthopaedic surgery that I should bring her to Dublin as she is a difficult patient to intubate. Listen to everything. Question everything. Be open to everything. There is not always a potential solution to a unique diagnosis or lack of diagnosis.

Nuggets for Millennials

Never underestimate the power of family and friends in a difficult situation. It is so empowering to have someone listen to you without judgment, without giving opinion and also tolerating the waterfall of tears that accompanies the conversation. Accept help when offered, be it a walk with a friend or a coffee or an invitation to dinner. It can be all too easy to shut yourself off from other people as the situation can seem lonely and, at times, does feel very isolating.

If your child gets a definitive diagnosis, look for a support group. These can be found online, through your consultant, public health nurse etc. I would absolutely involve your child in everyday activities as much as possible; talk to them, bring them for walks, car rides, for ice cream – whatever brings happiness to them and whatever makes the circumstances a little easier for both of you.

Do not hide your child away at home and always be open to answering questions about their condition if asked. From my experience, other children will ask 'what is wrong with.....?'And their parents often scold them for asking the question. I appreciate the openness of the questions from children. Whilst at a playground, a child asked me why my daughter was in a wheelchair so I explained that she was unable to walk and needed the wheelchair to get around. She looked puzzled and asked "

Why can't she walk?" so I explained that her muscles are weaker than those of other children and they 'Don't allow her to walk'. The young girl smiled and said 'Ok, I understand. I hope your muscles get stronger when you are older.' Some simple questions, followed by some simple answers.

If only we could look at each situation in such simple terms as children do. This would foster a greater sense of resilience in us all.

Brick by Brick

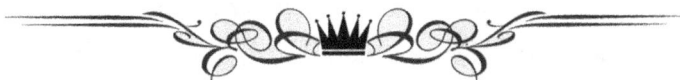

Mairtín O' HIobain

*"Remember, don't try to build the greatest wall
That's ever been built. Focus on laying a single,
expertly placed brick. Then keep doing that, every day".*

— Will Smith

To say that my earliest foundations in life were shaky, would be an understatement. My mother died when I was aged 5. The only memory I have of her, is that of her being carried down a hallway lined with my neighbours who came to see her before the funeral. I read an article recently (1) which gave the startling statistic that "2 in every 100, 9-year-olds in Ireland have lost a parent". Since I experienced such a major loss early in life, I was curious as to what the main effects on a child could be. It has been reported (2), that, children who experience parental loss are at a higher risk for many negative outcomes, including some of the following:

1. Mental issues (e.g., depression, anxiety, somatic complaints, post-traumatic stress symptoms),
2. Shorter schooling,
3. Less academic success,
4. Lower self-esteem (I used to be consumed by what others thought but this has lessened over the years)

Given the negative outcomes outlined above, it got me thinking about how my mum's death may have affected me as both a toddler and an adult. Could I relate to any of this? The short answer is a resounding yes.

After mum's passing, I spent a lot of time alone as a child and was sad for much of the time. Developing mental health issues was inevitable and a natural progression I suppose. My young mind had no coping strategies back then. Everything seemed so overwhelming. I have memories of endless days of going to school and mixing with other kids who seemed to have more than me in every way. Self-conscious thoughts scarred me early on in life. Thoughts like, why am I the only one without a mum and I couldn't accept my reality then. These comparisons intensified my sense of isolation. Growing up in a small house, in a large family, with money tight, life was tough.

My strongest memory of school was the week leading up to Mother's Day which was my worst nightmare. The teachers made us make Mother's Day cards every year. Having to do this, caused me huge anxiety. But it is also important to add that there were some good times too. My eldest sister stepped up to the plate and became mammy to us all.

I couldn't speak about my mum until recently. I suppose, writing this chapter opened- up a lot of old wounds, but it was important to confront them head on rather than keep them suppressed in my subconscious. Also, since becoming a parent, I have switched vantage points and it got me thinking about the unbearable emotional pain my mum must have gone through before her passing. Not seeing her kids again and not being there when they needed her the most. I have journeyed back to explore her life and found there were a lot of good times too. Being a new dad has helped me heal and brought a new empathy towards what she went through in her final days.

I left school at 14 and with little education to fall back on, I took the route of following my older brothers into the construction industry. I learnt my trade with one of my brothers and set up my own business at the young age of 22.

But with success, came large amounts of money, alcohol, and partying. I had bought three properties by 25 and was heading 'for the moon'. I achieved so much early on. Maybe the financial and emotional insecurity I experienced early in life, drove me on. I knew the only one that I could rely on back then was me, or so I thought. I was used to being self- reliant, more out of necessity than anything else.

Working for builders, who at the time seemed to have it all, led me to the false belief, that this was something I wanted to strive for. It seemed to be the Holy Grail, something to aspire to, and a measure of success and happiness. I was young and probably a bit inexperienced back then, unable to see what was right in front of me. It wasn't until many years later that I discovered that these men were living a lie and were no more than con men.

Then in 2008 the bubble burst and the Irish construction industry fell apart (3) and with it, the rental market. Ireland was facing an economic tsunami, a period of bust and bail outs. The storm clouds were gathering. With no education, no computer skills, and no jobs, I found myself sitting alone in my apartment, wondering, and worrying about what I was going to do to pay for three mortgages.

Prior to this hiatus, big bumps for me, were usually in the shape of a bad big night out or booze related, where that feeling of depression and hopelessness took weeks to clear. But, in time, at least they did clear. This situation was different, it was bigger, it was out of my control and I had no perceived way forward or way out. I found myself at a fork in the road with only 2 possible options – stay or emigrate.

From this feeling of hopelessness, I eventually found the inner strength to push myself forward and able to look at the other choices I may have. Who could I turn to for help/advice? I approached a friend who was living in Dublin and a man ahead of his time, and still is. He was sourcing work from an Internet referral site and convinced me to join him. From that, came a break in the form of a national insurer requiring an emergency building contractor. This led to a successful 14-year stint working with this insurer. Lady luck was finally shining on me. Blue sky at last!

So, I learned from this bump that having people to bounce your ideas off and open your mind to new opportunities is so important. Trying to go it alone, can be a lonely journey, especially when the challenges loom large.

The Insurance industry gave me the opportunity to upskill and to interact with professional people. My education came late in life, but in a timely fashion. This gave me my own insurance policy on myself and enabled me to generate an alternative income. I was building a portfolio of business options. I now had real choices.

Comeback Power

It is now roughly 20 years since I experienced those periods of my life when I was in a state of depression and despair, where my body would react physically and shutdown.

A long journey of learning and self-reflection followed which led me to the understanding of why and how one's mind can run wild and become the enemy lurking within. Choosing to attack at night when we are probably at our most vulnerable, depriving us of sleep and sanity.

Lessons I learnt about minding myself and building resilience

It is important to say at this juncture, that although I have learned these lessons, I sometimes forget to use them. Being human, we do our best!

- When running on empty, I look at ways to build my energy levels and recharge. At times like this, I seek some self -pampering, rather than increase my gym time. My wife and I go for regular spa treatments together.

- I remind myself daily of how grateful I am for the little diamonds I have in life and how lucky I am. "Gratitude can transform common days into thanksgiving, turn routine jobs into joy, and change ordinary opportunities into blessings." William Arthur Ward. This constant reminder keeps me optimistic and in a good emotional state during times of adversity.

- I now recognize those things which are out of my control. I realize that you can't affect other people's attitudes or actions, only your own. Put your energy into those things over which you have influence.

- I have learnt to forgive myself for the past. Indeed, the past is something over which you have no control. Learn from it and move on.

- I have built a strong support network of friends and family. As one of my favourite motivational speakers Les Brown says, "It is important to surround yourself with people who lift you up, encourage you, share your vision and inspire you". A key part of coping was to help others and spend time with family and friends. Make sure your friends know what you're thinking and be honest with them. They will see changes in you before you do. Also, by showing your vulnerability, you give them permission to do the same.

- I was so self-reliant, that I couldn't see that there were good people in my sphere who could help me when the going got rough. Reach out to trusted people in your circle and don't be afraid to seek their advice.

- Learn to become a better communicator making sure that you are being both heard and listened to equally.

- Give yourself time to grieve your losses and get professional support, if you need it, before the situation spirals out of control. Deal with life's issues early and don't give them power.

- I learned to take stock and make notes each time I went through a down period, which helped as a guide for the next time. It was a reference point and reminded me, that I had the ability to bounce back. Belief in this ability to recover, is 90% of the battle. I started looking at each setback as a setup for a comeback.

- Build a recovery folder with all your notes in one place to remind you how to deal with off days and bring you back from negative thought patterns.

- I put a family photo album on my phone and it is a great source of positive energy. Doing this will give you a lift when you need it most.

- Committing your thoughts and feelings to a journal can be a form of catharsis – out of your head and onto paper. It can be a fantastic stress relief valve during troubled periods and can be a reminder of how you found the strength to bounce back. What worked and what didn't.

- Keep a worry diary. It can be helpful to grant yourself permission to write out your problems for an allotted time each day (maybe 15 minutes) during times of increased stress. This is an anxiety reducing technique recommended by Leahy (4) in his book, 'The Worry Cure' – ask yourself the following questions:

    1. What am I worrying about?
    2. What am I feeling?
    3. What am I predicting?
    4. How much do I believe it will happen?
    5. What is the evidence for my prediction?
    6. What is the evidence against the prediction?

- Realize that most of the things we worry about will never happen

- Factor in down time to your day. A time where your brain can relax and switch off. For me it could be cooking or pottering in the garden.

- Have your own quiet space in the house where you can go and chill out or meditate. This could also be in your car.

- Let the child in you out to play. I love having play days with my daughter. She is a great little companion. I also enjoy goofing around with, my Maltese terrier. To see the world through my daughter's eyes has really helped me and I can relive my childhood. The joy she brings me is magic and to see her transition from a baby to a little person with her own character.

- An early walk in my garden is now the way I like to start my day, simply looking at nature and observing my thoughts rather than trying to control them.

- I listen to a 20min mediation in the morning before I go to work. I find, it's better to get up early and be prepared for whatever comes down the track.

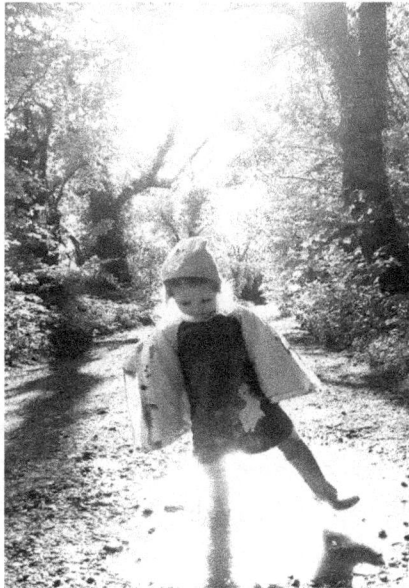

Lessons learned in business

- Don't put business ahead of your family life. You may get success but it will come at a price. Balance is key.

- Delegate – build a strong trustworthy team around you. Let them make mistakes and avoid the temptation to micromanage.

- Know when to step away from a deal if the cost is too great to your health.

- Play to your skills. Invest in your education if there is a piece of the jigsaw missing.

- Grow your portfolio, so that you have a plan B if one side of business goes belly up.

- Learn to say 'no' assertively, not aggressively. The ideal situation is when your business dealings come from a win/win place.

- Even if business failed in the past through bad dealings, learn the lessons and move on. The past doesn't define your future.

- Have people you can bounce your business ideas off and open your mind to new opportunities. Use some lateral thinking.

- Prioritize your time. Deal with the urgent and important things first.

- Find out what time of day works best for you. Maybe you work best in the morning and if so, assign your tough jobs to this time of day.

- Daily self -assessment – at the end of every day, ask yourself what worked and what needs improvement.

- Use technology – you don't have to drive everywhere to meet clients. You can use Teams, Zoom or Skype. There is also the option of meeting people half -way, so that the journey is halved for both of you. If, the Covid outbreak has taught us anything, it is how to manage the way we work.

Fast forward to 20/21

COVID-19 has grounded everyone, and this heightened sense of restriction is pushing people to their limits. Any insecurities which people may have, will be intensified in this unprecedented situation. All you need do, is turn on the news to get into the 'fear zone'. Most human contact is outlawed as we are all herded into our confined bubbles, and our daily lives have been turned upside down. Life has changed forever especially in the way we work. But this interruption to my working life has been a blessing in disguise for me, as I'm finally beginning to wake up and see that it's not all about working. It's spending time with my wife and daughter, that's what's important. The time I spend with them will give a new positive energy to deal with anything that may come my way.

I learned that in life, to quote an adage, one door closes, and another door opens. My takeaways based on my own hard learned lessons can be summarised below:

- If you have spare time, upskill. I got involved in smaller projects and learnt to be flexible working within the constraints of tighter budgets.

- There will be times when that black cloud will hover over you attempting to bring you down. You will repeatedly question your abilities. Belief in myself, has been my ongoing challenge. When it is quiet at work, I tend to freak out, telling myself I'm finished instead of being able to savour the down time. Put your thoughts in perspective, realizing that your past doesn't define your future. I reverse my thinking by concentrating on all the things I have achieved, rather than those I haven't.

- One of my biggest regrets was working excessively and missing my daughters first year of life. As I said, being quiet at work is torture for me and it makes me believe I'm going to lose everything when logic tells me, that I am also in one of the few industries that expands in times of recession. I now have balance in my life, family, and work in harmony. As Goethe says, *"Things that matter most must never be at the mercy of things that matter least".*

- I can be a bit of a slob to live with, so, I try to pull my weight and help with cleaning once a week, and invariably cooking at the weekend so that my wife can go for a walk.

- Being outside in the garden is one of the great joys in my life. I am in the process of converting my garage into a home office which will allow me to work from home more often, freeing up time to spend with my family and in the garden. Working in the garden and on home projects feeds my drive for work thus keeping my mind active and sane. We spend lots of time outside together. Real dad/daughter bonding time – heaven!

Walking in the wilderness, rudderless for a period following an involuntary change of direction in your life, can be part of your life's journey. Plotting your next move can often be difficult during these periods as it reminds you of the events that led you to this juncture in the past. There will be all sorts of mixed feelings. But time can be a great healer and teacher.

Negative thoughts surrounding the trauma which triggered these feelings will always be nearby trying to invade your mind with doubts attempting to pull you down. And there may be physical manifestations of these feelings.

By consciously halting and challenging this negative recursive loop playing out in your mind, you begin to take back your power. Think of these thoughts as if in a court case. Ask yourself what evidence there is to support these negative feelings of insecurity now. As I play this out in my mind, I realize how much I have grown in the last few years and how much I have achieved in moving forward. My foundations are much stronger now. I have the tools to cope. I am not the insecure young man I was in my 20s, I am a lot more assertive and confident with a strong support system in place. I also recognise the signals when I need my down time and what nourishes my being.

These positives and negatives must be viewed in a certain light. If we can have negative thoughts, it also stands to reason that the opposite is true. So, on balance its 50/50. The pendulum swings both ways. Once you accept this, you are halfway there. This mind-set will give you a real boost. It will help build your resilience in times of adversity.

To learn to breathe slowly through my nose was invaluable when situations of concern arose and helped me to slow down. If, you can't see how lucky you are, then allow life to show you. To be content with where you are in life and especially with times of good health. We stress about relatively small things in life and make them into monsters which torture us.

But sometimes it takes a paradigm shift to make you see that what you worry about can be dwarfed very easily. Recently, my friend told me about his son's friend who has fallen ill and has been taken out of child- care. This boy is the same age as my daughter Holly. In telling me about this sad story, I could sense that it took a lot out of him. I also felt the sadness. All the money and success in the world means nothing when a child is seriously ill.

To appreciate your family's good health, as there are family's that pray for good health.

Your foundations will get stronger. Be patient with yourself and focus on laying a single expertly placed brick. Then keep doing that every day.

*I wish to thank my ghost writer, Giselle Marrinan, who worked closely with me in the telling of my story.

References

(1) Lynch, P. "Children Living with Loss" earlychildhoodireland.ie, 13th Nov 2018.

(2) "How Does the Death of a Parent Affect a Child"? www.parentingforbrain.com. Feb 22nd, 2021.

(3) McDonald, F. "The Fall of the Mighty Developers" The Irish Times, 12th June 2009.

(4) Leahy, R.L. "The Worry Cure; Stop Worrying and Start Living" Piatkus Books, 2006

Through the Mist: Faith, Friendship and Freedom

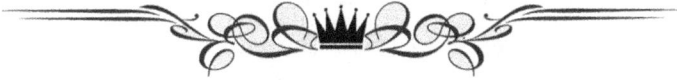

Mary Leroy

"Stop acting so small.
You are the universe in ecstatic motion"

— Rumi

hy did Rumi's quote speak so loudly to me? And what did it have to do with my life? Well, let's start with my interpretation of it. My belief is that we all have skills and talents no matter what our situation in life. Whether able bodied or disabled. We can all contribute something to the world if only to hold up a mirror to others. We are constantly moving, changing and evolving. I was challenged with a life changing event in my 20s and as a result, I could have crawled into a corner and stayed there. But a small voice inside me kept pushing me on and I am so glad that I listened. By acting small, my life would have shrunk and I would never have become the person I am today; had the adventures I have had or enjoyed the love I found throughout my adult life. So, here is my story warts and all. I hope it encourages you to expand like the universe into the beauty and wonder of you. Your footprint in this world is unique and special!

I grew up in 1960s Lancashire, in what can best be described as something from a Catherine Cookson novel, with cruel rich men and innocent poor girls and rags-to-riches careers and melodramatic loves and hates.

Mary Leroy

My family went from having money to poverty. My dad was brought up with a 'golden spoon' but had no idea how to manage wealth. He was left a 100-acre farm by his father when he was married and turned twenty-one but had no skills on the day to day running of it, so in time lost everything through lack of knowledge and poor management. What little money he had, would be spent on buying locals drinks in the bar or luxuries he could ill afford. He was forced to file for bankruptcy when he was 30 because of his poor decisions and because his sisters complained that they hadn't got their share of the profits from the family farm. With a young family of 5 children and my mum to care for, he became a gardener when I was seven and worked for Heinz as a cleaner to make ends meet.

He was a controlling man who literally ruled his family with an iron fist. The violence started when I was two. He physically and mentally tortured my mother and we learnt from an early age not to cross him. If you were wise, you would stay clear of him. So, my earliest feelings were those of fear and insecurity. Not unsurprisingly, I became wary of men from an early age but thought that all families were like this. I didn't know any different.

I left home at eighteen on a scholarship to study social sciences at university. But my father insisted I come home every weekend so he could keep a close eye on me. It was part of his controlling nature. I learned later in life that he was proud of the fact that I went to university. When my father died of a massive heart attack at just fifty-three, I came home to be near my mother as she had developed cancer.

Since my mother was a very insecure person who also tried to gently steer my life, I ended up getting my own flat nearby with my friend Sally. I guess I needed to individuate now that I had the freedom of being away to study. Sally and I both worked in the same field and were going to go on further courses to improve our skills. Little did I know what lay in wait for me. In the words of John Lennon, *"Life is what happens while you are busy making other plans"*.

The occasion of my twenty-fourth birthday was a day like no other. This was a significant day in so many ways. The day when my life as I knew it changed forever, the day I had a stroke which left me partially paralyzed.

It was a day that could have defined the rest of my life had it not been for the intervention of Peter, a person who up onto that point had been on the periphery of my life. But let me back up a little.

After this life–changing event, I lost all confidence in myself. My then boyfriend disappeared unable to cope with my disability. In the hospital, I could see and hear people, but I became trapped in my own head, because initially, I was unable to communicate with those around me. I could understand them, but they couldn't understand me. I had total paralysis down the right-hand side of my body, general weakness, and the use of only my non-dominant left hand. My face was also paralysed down one side making me look like someone akin to Quasimodo. This was a surreal experience. I had never been so disconnected from life.

Apparently, everyone around me was expecting my imminent death and couldn't look me straight in the eye for fear, I could read their thoughts. The doctors spoke over me, saying that death was inevitable after a stroke like mine and people at my bedside were encouraging me to 'cross over'. I heard every word but couldn't speak to say that I was fighting to stay alive. I listened to everyone because I wasn't strong enough to do anything else. I had to accept death if that was to come. Interesting though, those who were close to me, said that during this time, that they could tell from my eyes that I was still in there somewhere.

The knowledge that I might die in hospital was terrifying, but I also knew that I wasn't alone there. I had another partner inside me who was totally supporting me. It was like an echo of a small voice. It was making more sense than those words uttered around the bed. It simply said, "I will be with you". It wasn't promising that I would live, but rather that no matter what happened, I wasn't alone. To me it was God, my higher self, the universe. At that young age, it was difficult to know or name who was rooting for me. All I knew was that I had to accept where I was being led and let go trying to control the next step.

Up to the age of eighteen, I played a strong role in the church and worked closely with our vicar. However, at University I questioned everything. I was a little at sea and became ambivalent to what I saw as 'religiosity'. It didn't help, the fact that one day, the vicar I had known so well on leaving the bedside of someone he had come to visit, just nodded in my direction, and left. He made no attempt to speak to me.

My faith was to become stronger further down the line, roughly nine years later.

Knowledge of the fact that I was in the minority, rooting for myself, I knew I had to make a plan. I must welcome life whilst I was still in it and enjoy the special moments when I could.

My first mission should I accept it, was to make myself understood. So, I had to make use of whatever I had in my limited state. I couldn't talk and although I could read, I couldn't comprehend what anything I was reading was about. I used to turn away if there were too many people around me or just sit and listen and hope they would go away.

In fact, I realised that I needed to help people as much as I could to get them to understand me. People when they are sat with a warm person who is not able to respond can tell you a lot. And I learnt a lot about their personal lives. Things that maybe they wouldn't have told me if I had been able to respond. That made me feel useful. I was their' private sounding board. I chuckled a bit at the unwitting knowledge about their personal lives which they freely volunteered.

I still resisted leaving my hospital space until I had to. Eventually the decision was made for me by the staff. I was pushed outside into the quadrangle because I was in a very elderly ward and having people dying is some-what difficult both for a twenty something patient and indeed my visitors. Unbeknownst to me, there were bigger plans for my life. I couldn't remain the caterpillar hiding in my cocoon.

I was sat in the quadrangle one very hot summer's day with no hat. There was nothing in this quadrangle except for tiles. Then the door opened and out came my sister, Margaret. Her mother in law and a swiftly moving exuberant five-year-old niece.

Before anybody could stop her, she had climbed up onto the wheel of my wheelchair, looked me straight in the eyes and said, "Are you going to have a baby or are you going to die?" Both ladies jumped up and my niece was shuttled off to the car. I just burst out laughing. Not only was it the first time anybody had made me laugh, but it was also the first time that people acknowledged that there was a difficulty. My niece had unwittingly made it acceptable to talk to me directly and get a response. I was grateful for that. Out of the mouths of babes!!

This was a turning point for all. It was safe to talk about 'It'.

After two months, I was released from hospital. I was able to return home, this time to live with my mum. But all the plans I had to further my education stopped. My world fell silent again and I resisted meeting people because of my speech problems which were still quite severe.

Because of my disability, people would speak to me through my mum, "Do you think Mary would like some cake?". Very hard to take when you are still the intelligent grown up inside but can't communicate to the outside world. It was as if I had left the planet and was somewhat invisible. This made me curl up and want to isolate even more from people. As, Rumi said, I was acting small to protect myself and stay safe. I had a language impairment, a condition known as chronic aphasia. I thought if I battened down the hatches, then I could live in my own little world.

Mary Leroy

The Kindness of Strangers

I was soon to learn about the kindness of people. People who were peripheral to my life. In the 1970s, my world collided with a person I can only describe now, as my 'twin soul'. Peter worked in the administration department of social services. I used to call him when I was a social worker requesting forms but hadn't ever met him. He was three foot six inches but never let this impediment interfere with his enjoyment of life. On the contrary, he became stronger because of and despite his challenge. It was his personality you noticed first and foremost. He heard through the grapevine, that I was holed up in my parent's house, refusing to engage with people and indeed the outside world, he acted decisively.

He arrived out to the farmhouse and requested an audience with me. No softly, softly approach with him. Peter was direct and to the point. During our conversation, he challenged me with these statements, "I am here because you can get into a car"; "You have a disability, deal with it".

He then announced that we were going to the local pub. This wasn't a question, but more along the lines of an implied command. There was no debate around this decision and no reasonable argument that could be made in protest. So off we trotted together in his car. Can you imagine the scene as we entered the normally loud and raucous country pub.

As the door swung open, there was me leaning on a stick, heart pounding and my vertically challenged companion standing in the doorway. The place fell silent. It was like a scene from one of those old spaghetti Westerns. As we made our way to the bar, we started laughing uncontrollably. Two partners in crime. This was my first tentative move out of the mist and into the real world. In the words of the author Mary Radmacher (1) *"Courage doesn't always roar. Sometimes courage is the little voice at the end of the day that says I'll try again tomorrow"*

Happenstance or A Hidden Hand in My Life?

This was to be the first of many significant and hidden moves in my life. You could call it happenstance, but I know that there has been a bigger hand nudging me forward, one tentative step at a time. My second husband Richard was a 6- foot handsome detective who to the outside world seemed like a big cuddly personable guy. We were married for 9 years and for the first few years, things were good between us. After a while, certain traits in him began to come to the fore. He became jealous around me and more controlling, trying to keep me in a figurative 'Ivory Tower'. He started waking me up at 3 in the morning asking me to tell him what I had been up to that day and trying to trip me up on details. I felt like I was on high alert constantly having to defend myself. I became one of his cases.

Towards the end of our marriage, he became more violent. I would wake up to find his hands around my throat. The final straw came, when I had to go to Portugal on a work trip to accompany a group of disabled people and their carers. Richard was really angry that I had decided to go away. So much so, that I was going to cancel the trip until the travel company announced that they needed a certain number of carers to qualify for the safety flight requirements. My attendance was pivotal. When I returned to London, I discharged my duty with the group and instead of going home, made my way in the evening straight to Waterloo station. I knew I had to keep going and escape from my marriage. I truly believed that had I returned home, in time Richard would have killed me.

I vividly recall this incident at Waterloo station in London, a day when I was distraught. I was running away from Richard, brow beaten and terrified and needed to make a call to my friend Sally in Salisbury to tell her I was coming to stay.

I went to the ticket desk with what I thought was 20 pounds and a 10p but realized that my money was all in foreign coins. Realizing my dismay, the chap at the kiosk told me to just give him what I had. How often does this happen! Armed with my ticket, I realized that I now had no change to phone my friend – the last part of my great escape was about to fall apart. At this point, a Scotsman standing on the platform called me over and on handing me 10p, asked me to phone his wife to tell her, he was on his way home. Just as I turned, he shouted after me "Forget it, I just realized that she is staying with our daughter tonight". He had disappeared before I could return his money. Now I had 10p to phone my friend. Two angels came to my rescue that day in my hour of need!

Finding 'The One'

It took two marriage breakdowns before I met Gerard and found love at last. People think, including myself in the past, that one can't find love if you have a disability. Making friends is probably the only option available to you. I am here to tell you that this isn't true.

My first marriage to a Scottish guy called Andrew lasted all of 3 months. The marriage itself lasted a few years but I legally left it after a few months. I came from a wealthy family and he decided, since his circumstances were poor to target me. I guess when he asked me to marry him, I thought it would be a good route to a 'normal life' after my stroke. Shortly after our marriage, he started contacting my family looking for money, explaining that things were hard for him the way I was. I was on a good salary at the time and because we had a joint account, he was able to drain it. He left taking all the money and the furniture. Before I met Gerard, both of my previous marriages had come from a place of 'wanting to be normal'. They didn't come from a place of deep love and respect.

Gerard found me when I wasn't looking. He literally bumped into me at a busy Sunday market. I was walking with a heavy knapsack and a drunk man fell into my path and landed hard on the ground. I sidestepped to miss him and lost my footing. This stranger (Gerard) grabbed my arm to steady me and he had this wonderful ability to calm me down. He was so kind and caring. We talked for a while and ended up sitting on a beach in Southend chatting for hours. And as the saying goes, 'The rest is history'.

Meeting Gerard was one of the most beautiful events of my life. I had no idea, that the day he grabbed my arm in the market, was to be the day that changed my life forever. It took another five years before we married as I had developed a mistrust of relationships, but our friendship blossomed into something deeper. Although he was 17 years older than me, none of this mattered. I had reached a safe harbour and the love we found together was deep and profound

He is an encourager and supporter, but that doesn't mean that he doesn't challenge me to push the boundaries. He sees ME, and that my disabilities are just a part, not all of me. I always wanted to travel the world and he made sure to make my dream come true in spades. If someone helps you to become a better person, then hold on tight.

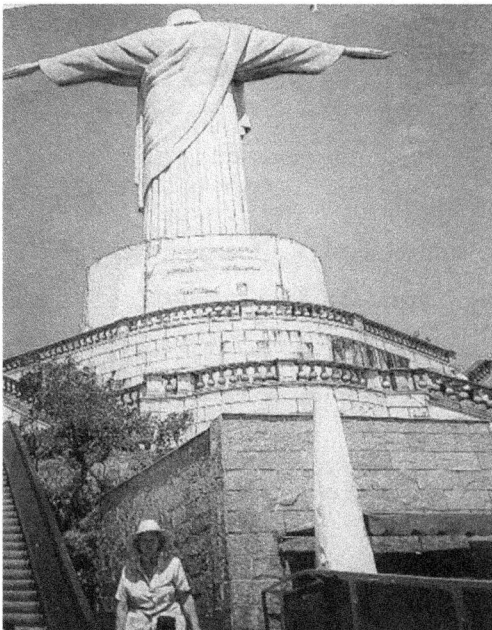

Let Your Life Speak

Elizabeth Fry (2) certainly reflected the saying, 'Let your lives speak', meaning let your lives reflect your values. I respected this value of veering away from a duplicitous life, as many people say one thing and do another. It was something I could aspire to and respect. Since speech had been a struggle for me for so long, the idea of being heard and understood by a community also spoke to me. The small voice which I spoke of in hospital, was at last finding the space and silence in which to be heard. When I walked into my first 'Friends Meeting' (3), I just knew I was at home. I craved the silence that I found. It was my safe place. A place to grow and explore without a tranche of rules. It was my spiritual 'base camp'.

I still struggled to hear God. It seemed like He had gone quiet even though I had at last found my spiritual home. So, I went on a retreat in 1993 when I was 42, just before Easter. It was here that I encountered the 'two wise men' who were our leaders whilst we were there. I remember saying to them that I thought that God had stopped talking to me. One of the leaders said, "Just give me a picture of you and God". I replied, "I see God and myself sitting quietly side by side in front of a roaring fire and instinctively knowing that He is there". At this point the second leader who was a bit of a recluse piped in with, "What do you want"? To which I retorted, "I want a conversation with Him". He took a few minutes of reflection and said in a quiet voice, "The silence and not the tittle tattle of conversation, is where two people who feel comfortable with each other are able to be. That is precious".

This was the eureka moment of faith for me. I had my answer at last. I was expecting God on tap when He was sitting beside me all along. Like the song I had heard on U Tube some years back sung by a 10- year old blind autistic boy Christopher, "Open the Eyes of My Heart". (4) My spiritual heart was now reawakened.

Lessons Learned

- Trust in the goodness of strangers.

- Don't let it your disability stop you travelling and fulfilling your passion of seeing different countries. With Gerard's help, I walked some of the Great Wall of China, travelled to Brazil, Nagasaki, Italy, France, Mauritius, Kruger Park in South Africa, Australia, South America, Israel, Turkey, Egypt, and Russia. Also, I still want to go to the Galápagos Islands.

- What appears to others to be happenstance, I know to be part of a bigger move in our lives showing us that we are not alone.

- Learn to laugh at yourself. Humour has been identified as a possible factor in the development of personal resilience (5). It took a 5-year-old to teach me how to laugh again. I also recall my friend Sally saying to me after returning from hospital, "Well I guess this stops your chances of becoming an air hostess".

- Don't worry if you make a mistake (as in my first two marriages), you can always go back to the drawing board.

- Listen to other's advice but ultimately make decisions for yourself based on your own inner strength and belief-your higher self.

- Find out what makes you happy. I love chocolate, sitting looking at nature, cuddling up in bed and many other things which nourish me.

- Identify at least one person in your life who you can turn to if everything falls apart. Someone who won't judge you but will hold a safe place for you until you can find your wings and fly again.

- It has been said of me, that I am very sure of who I am now. My beliefs, ethos, indeed my sense of what's right and wrong are something I hold strongly to today. It may make me unpopular at times but if I am not me, not congruent, then who am I? People can take me or leave me, it's their choice. As Oscar Wilde once said, "*Be yourself, everyone else is taken*"

- If you find faith/ belief in something greater than yourself or rediscover it later in life, hold on fast. Pursue your 'safe place'. A place which aligns with your values. Regardless of what you believe in, know that someone is there fighting in your court. My reawakening has withstood the test of time and is now pivotal to my life. It has been my strength. I leave you with the key. question I asked the participants of a workshop I ran with some colleagues in 2009. **What would you like your life to say?**

*I wish to thank my ghost writer, Giselle Marrinan, who worked closely with me in the telling of my story.

References

(1) Radmacher, M.A. "Courage Doesn't Always Roar" Conari Press March 2009

(2) christianity.org.uk/article/elizabeth-fry

(3) www.bbc.co.uk/religion/religions/christianity/subdivisions/quakers_1.shtml

(4) www.youtube.com/watch?v=wPTMA7HIIyk

(5) "Why It's Incredibly Important to Learn to Laugh at Yourself" www.huffpost.com. Dec   6th, 2017

Eldrick

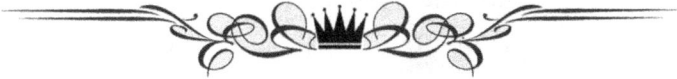

Ray Flannery

I can hear some of you ask just exactly who or what is an Eldrick? and more importantly, what has this to do with RESILIENCE. To make things easier for any person who has no interest in sport or more specifically an interest in the world of golf, or who has just emerged from the rock they have been living under, let me explain. If I don't, the title of my chapter will have no meaning whatsoever for them. For those people I will refer to Eldrick by his globally known alternative name…TIGER. Yes, the person I would like to base my chapter on, is the one and only Eldrick Tont "Tiger" Woods. In my opinion, this man is the absolute definition of resilience. I can hear some of you questioning this because Tiger Woods is a phenomenally successful sportsman, who for many years seemed to be absolutely unbeatable. The one person on the planet who had both the talent, mindset, and age on his side to finally surpass the legend that is Jack Nicklaus in his winning of eighteen Majors. To date, this has not come to fruition. YET!

Let's roll the clock back a few years. Eldrick Woods was born on the 30th of December 1975. His father Earl was a retired U.S. Army officer who met his wife Kultida in Thailand in 1968 when he was deployed there. Earl introduced Tiger to the game of golf before he was two years old. The fact that Earl was in the Army allowed the young Tiger to go to courses owned by the military to practice. In 1978 Tiger had his first TV appearance putting against the legendary comedian Bob Hope. At the age of just eight, Tiger won the 9-10 boys' event at the Junior World Golf Championship. The prodigy's light was starting to shine. The first obstacle in the world of Tiger Woods started to raise its ugly head around this time…RACISM. Unbelievably there were certain courses that the rising star was not welcomed to tee it up at, simply due to the fact that he was a person of colour. In some people's eyes this young athlete had no business attending the facilities that their large bank balances or place in society afforded them the opportunity to become members.

The next factor that crept into the life of the young Tiger Woods was plain and simple JEALOUSY. There were a lot of other players around this time who had served their times on the various tours without ever becoming successful. Now here was this kid setting foot in their backyard and playing their game his way. Tiger had the skill at a very young age to simply hit the ball further, more accurately and more consistently than they could ever imagine. It was also at this time that Tiger started to gain notoriety amongst the golfing elite. This seemingly God given talent was so much given as earned though. Earl Woods was a tough task master who had orchestrated the young Tiger's fledgling career with military precision. Earl had sneakily put plans into place to have Tiger coached by the current best coaches on the circuit. Earl was ruthless, he lied, harassed, cajoled these coaches into taking a very active part in the career of the prodigy. Hours and hours of practice were put in by Tiger, all within the earshot of Earl. The downside of this practise was the lack of a normal childhood being enjoyed by Tiger. A sacrifice which, in the mind of Earl Woods was going to be worth every millisecond of lost time playing silly games with the other kids. DETERMINATION… The will to succeed and at the same time please his taskmaster father in my mind, are two of the driving forces which led to the determination which has been continuously shown by Tiger throughout his golfing career. If Earl was happy, then Tiger was happy. They say that if you find a job that you love then you will never work a day in your life. In the case of Tiger Woods I am not one hundred per cent sure if this is the case. As a golfer, and I say that in the loosest of terms, I struggle to practice a few times a month. To practice those drills for six or seven hours every day along with attending school and studying demonstrates a level of resilience that only very few can match. Along the way there were a few setbacks, as one would expect but the mantras instilled into the brain of Tiger by Earl would prove enough to get him through.

The success enjoyed by Tiger brought with it the obvious rewards. The college places offered, the endorsements, the contracts though were all masterminded by Earl. At only twenty-one years of age, Tiger became the youngest ever Master's champion and in doing so winning by the largest ever margin in the tournament's history. I will not however start to list all of the victories and achievements which can be attributed to Tiger Woods or else this entire volume would be Tiger's career statistics and nothing else, except to say that in the next decade Tiger would go on to win thirteen of his fifteen Majors. The next decade would paint a different landscape. A series of personal issues married with a list of injuries took its toll on the career of Tiger. All was not rosy in the garden of Tiger Woods. Tiger had married Elin Nordegren, a Swedish former model in 2004. Six years later Tiger and Elin were divorced. Rumours of extramarital affairs had surfaced and were denied in November 2009. Only a few days after these rumours surfaced, Tiger was involved in a collision in his SUV near his home. Initially the injuries were only superficial but then actually ruled him out of playing a charity tournament in which Tiger was the host. As the weeks passed, several more women came forward with claims of affairs. The result of the infidelities and injuries forced Tiger to announce that he would be taking an indefinite break from golf. However, the far reaching result of these admissions caused several companies to re-examine their association with one of the most recognisable faces on the planet. Now don't get me wrong, this man was never going to be short of a few quid but it wasn't only the loss of these multi-million endorsements that were going to be affected. His golfing status slumped. His surgery count started to mount, from possible career ending knee and back surgeries. The one time king of the golfing world was now snowballing downhill at a serious rate of knots.

In 2017, Tiger was arrested for driving under the influence of alcohol or drugs. His mugshot appeared globally on every sort of social and print media available. There was going to be no way back from this. Every sports journalist had written his epitaph. The King was no more. That same year Tiger had undergone his fourth back surgery, his career ranking was 1,199. He had even admitted to his friends that he "was done". The dreams of equalling the 18 Majors was over. The intense rehab needed after the various surgeries, tied in with the hiring and firing of different coaches, his firing of his caddy Steve Williams, the affairs, the arrests, the substance abuse looked like signalling the end.

Amazingly though, someone forgot to give that note to Tiger. The rehab was starting to pay off and not just the physical type. Tiger started yet another comeback in March 2018, after a few near misses, Tiger presented himself in his familiar attire of red top and black trousers in the winners' circle at East Lake Golf Club. On the 14th of April 2019, Eldrick Tiger Woods won his first Major championship in eleven years which brought his total of major wins to fifteen, the scenes of the swathing crowds walking behind Tiger on the final few holes in Augusta Golf Club still send shivers down my spine. To have overcome all that, he has had to endure, albeit some of them self-inflicted, in my opinion is the very definition of resilience. I truly thought that I was going to witness somebody overhaul the 18 Major milestone, at least I did until the 23rd of February 2021, when Tiger was involved in a serious car crash which resulted in multiple leg injuries and surgery for non-life-threatening injuries. It is unclear as to when or even if Tiger Woods will grace the first tee of another Major tournament. I for one sincerely hope he does. This is probably going to be one of the toughest tests of resilience ever but, if there is anybody on the planet who can see a way of achieving this feat it is ELDRICK TIGER WOODS.

From the Archives:

Book Chapters on Resilience from Book Hub
Publishing Publications

THE Doc Check
Research, Consulting & Bespoke Training

Brokenness, a Prerequisite to Resilience?

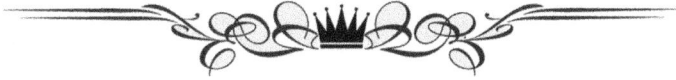

Giselle Marrinan

From the Book 'Calling You Connecting With A Life Coach of 25 Years' (Book Hub Publishing, 2020).

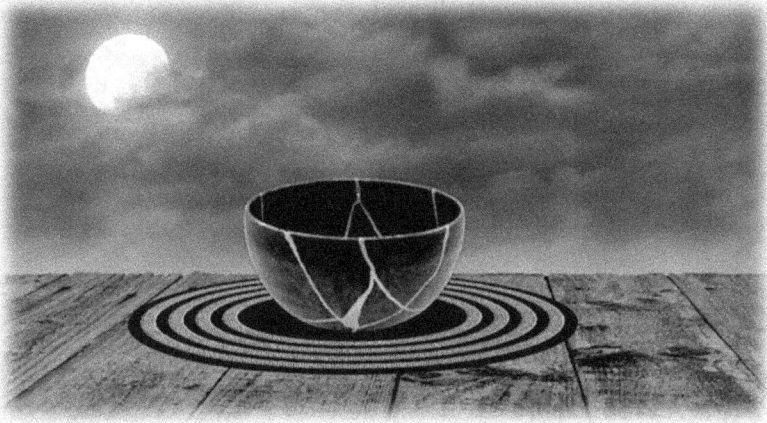

I n Japanese culture, broken objects are often lovingly repaired with gold. The flaw is seen as a unique and special part of the object's history hence adding to its beauty. Perhaps something to consider when you feel broken.

Recently, whilst driving from Edinburgh to catch the ferry to Belfast, I happened upon an interview on BBC radio Scotland with an 81-year-old cyclist called Mavis Paterson. Her story is incredible and a real testament to how resilience can be borne from tragedy and brokenness. I have listed the salient points from the interview below, but you may wish to research this lady further:

- She is officially the oldest women to have recently cycled the 960 miles from Land's End in western Cornwall to John O'Groats in the extreme northern point of mainland Scotland.
- She must go into hospital soon for hip and knee replacements. She has osteoarthritis and is in a lot of pain whilst walking
- She has raised more than £75,000 for Macmillan Cancer Support
- When she was 70, she cycled across Canada
- For her 80th birthday two years ago, she cycled for 24 hours
- She lost her 3 children all in their 40s

How does she keep going you may ask yourself? I think the clue is in something she said," I always set myself a goal and a challenge and it takes my mind off the grief that I suffer with losing my children"

By my reckoning, we have two choices when loss knocks us sideways. We can stay in the ensuing sadness and grief or we can pick ourselves up and find meaning in the life we have left. I speak from experience here. Over the last 3 years, I have lost my older brother, my 3 aunts and mum in quick succession. Sure, I went through the grief and sense of loss and still have moments of acute sadness, but I decided to put my energy into writing my first book (1), 'Another Zero', which I dedicated to my mum. She died in February, and my book was launched in November of the same year.

I am not by any means saying, that we all deal with loss in the same way, but what I am saying, is that it is good to develop some resilience/coping mechanisms sooner rather than later. If it's one sure thing about life, over time, we will be blindsided by something unforeseen and totally out of our control.

How are Millennials Coping with Today's Pandemic World?

In a report in Forbes (2) last year, a survey of young millennials undertaken by Deloitte, reported that a quarter of young millennials had lost their job or were placed on temporary unpaid leave due to the pandemic. But surprisingly, in 11 of the 13 countries, respondents, contrary to their situation, reported lower levels of stress. So, what is going on? Although they have been deeply affected by the changes in the world, they seem to have a sense of optimism about playing an active part in setting the global reset button.

Their hope for a better world is encouraging. They are looking for ways to improve society and want to be part of the solution. They are looking for ways to encourage businesses and governments to become more accountable to society.

Furthermore, an encouraging three fourths of those surveyed said, "the pandemic has made them more sympathetic toward others' needs and that they will take actions to have a positive impact on their communities in the future".

I think their hope and sense of altruism is helping to keep them resilient in the face of adversity. A lesson to us all. Without hope and the will to become part of the solution, we all feel powerless.

So how can we start building resilience? I have taken some tips from my book, 'Another Zero' which may help address the issue:

Building Resilience

- Make a simple decision today, of how you can begin to change your toxic thinking. This could begin with, something as simple as: giving those you meet, the benefit of the doubt. Innocent until proven guilty! Just because someone you know passes you by without waving, doesn't mean they are necessarily ignoring you. It could be they are preoccupied.

- Ask yourself: Why you need to hold on to old patterns of thought and behaviour. How is it benefitting your life? When we repeatedly stimulate a 'circuit' in the brain, we strengthen it. So, make sure to trigger as many positive thoughts and memories as possible.

- Let go of the need to control and possess things and people. I saw a quote from Saint John of The Cross, which summarized this point beautifully: *"There is a freedom in a love which does not have glue on its hands: it brings more joy, more refreshment; this joy just cannot happen in a person who is possessively caught up"*.

- Develop, the *'then what?'* pattern of thinking (taken from the field of REBT – rational emotive behavioural therapy). If you tend to worry, ask yourself: *"What is the worst thing that could happen?"* Chances are, in most scenarios, it won't be as bad as you thought.

In a company, for which I worked years ago, I remember playing out this scenario with the finance officer. For every fear, he voiced, I repeated: *"And then what?"* He started with his fear of sales decreasing; then budgets not being met; then finally, the fact that jobs would be cut with the ensuing inevitability of staff losses. When he had burnt himself out, with every negative scenario he could envisage, I said to him: *"If you lost your job, you would have more time to go fishing"* (knowing that this was his secret passion in life). He stopped dead in his tracks and looking intensely at me, his face changed from a grimace, to a smile and eventually a laugh. Worry defused! As it turns out, things weren't as gloomy as he had depicted, and everyone kept their job. Lesson learned!

The next time you or someone in your circle starts to worry about something that may happen, try out this technique. Keep going until you unearth the worst-case scenario. What is the outcome you or your friend fear most?

- Beware of the language you are using to and about yourself. For example: you could be using the word *'always'* just a little bit too often. Look for evidence in your life to counter statements that begin with always e.g. "I always suck at relationships". You might have a great friend for years, so this isn't true and so on.

- When something bad happens, don't react immediately. Give yourself a few minutes to think about the best response. In most cases, according to psychologist Jennifer Delgado: We have an *'emotional hijack'* (also coined as an amygdala hijack, by Daniel Goleman) when we act too quickly, due to being carried away by our feelings. If this happens, we tend to do or say something which we later regret. If you doubt the seriousness of the repercussions of this, consider the famous fight in 1993 where the boxer Mike Tyson bit off part of Evander Holyfield's ear. Some people believe the former's action, occurred because he reacted too quickly, for fear of losing his title; thus, bypassing the brains emotional filter, the amygdala. His mistake is purported to have cost him $3 million dollars and his boxing licence. *Always think first!* The power of emotions can overtake our rationality.

- Be mindful of what you are letting in through your eye and ear gates. Things like the news, negative documentaries showing the seedy underbelly of society, or gratuitously violent and sexually explicit movies, can have a deep-seated influence over our subconscious mind. Subliminal messages can seriously affect your way of thinking. They tend to cover 5 main topics: sex, fear, drugs, food, and violence. Dale Archer has cited many studies on violent video games. They have shown that, if the brain is repeatedly exposed to these, eventually the person will lose touch with reality and may even increase hostile behaviour. Be careful of life's hypnotists!

- Think of someone you really respect, either in your social circle or beyond. Ask yourself how they cope with tough challenges? What can you learn from them?

- Come to terms with failure. We all fail now and again. See it as strength. If we didn't fail, how else could we learn? They say: when you fall off a horse, you should get back up immediately (Trust me, I know this is true).

"Happiness is like a beautiful wild animal, watching from the edge of a forest. If you try to grab it, it will run away. But if you sit by your campfire and add some sticks to it, happiness will come to you and stay"

— Rick Hanson

- Take time out of each day, to meditate / pray. Get into a routine of giving the brain a rest. There are more ways to communicate with us than ever before. Unfortunately, this can distract us from what is important. So, we need to take time to go inward and away from distractions

- Have some quiet periods scheduled into your day. Since I stopped my crazy busy lifestyle, I now, thanks to my age and where I find myself in life, have more time to commune with nature. One of my favourite occupations is observing the birds, on my walks. Fellow Belfastonian, Robert Lynd says: *"In order to see birds, it is necessary to become a part of the silence"*. Is this also true of life in general? No matter what age we are, or whatever our circumstances, we must be silent now and again to absorb and engage in our precious life.

I recently watched a Ted Talk, given by the novelist, Pico Iyer on 'The Art of Stillness in an Accelerated life'. His recommendation of: *"Taking a few minutes out of every day, to recall what moves you most and where your truest happiness lies"*, stood out and caught my attention. If you don't know the answer, isn't it worth dedicating some time out of your life to find out?

"Sometimes making a living and building a life, point in opposite directions"

— Pico Iyer

- When you catch yourself using the words: "I can't", at least investigate the evidence behind this statement. I always compare this to being a barrister in court; bring the evidence for and against your case. If the facts don't stack up, revisit your original statement. Somewhere, your beliefs about yourself and your own abilities may be flawed.

- Don't let one bad experience determine your path in life. You are bigger than that. Use the lessons learned, to move on and maybe help others. If you need professional help, then seek it.

- Surround yourself with people who affirm you as a person. We have all seen what physical assaults can do because the results are obvious. However, this is worth noting: when people hurt us with abusive language and negative statements, researchers have found that the *same area* of the brain, (known as the cingulate gyrus) is impacted as when, we are physically injured. In other words, the pain is similar, meaning that physical and emotional pain, have similar neural signatures. Knowing this fact, will make you more mindful of those people, with whom you have chosen to spend most of your time.

- Make a list of all your good points. Some people say there is nothing good about themselves and feel quite embarrassed to be asked to do this task. Remember this is your secret list. At first this may be foreign to you. Start off with something tiny and build on this. This will develop resilience and will be helpful on days when your confidence takes a nosedive.

- Start a positive book. Keep a record of all the notes, cards and positive texts, emails etc. that anyone has ever said about and to you. You may also want to write in memories of special days, moments, and occasions in your life where you felt truly alive and free. You may want to stick in pictures of people who make you smile. Whatever you choose to include is up to you. With one proviso! It must be positive!

"Like the Tuatha De Danann, I will turn sideways towards the light, to avoid conversations that will make me a smaller person"

— David Whyte

Final Thoughts

What pieces of gold make up the fabric of your life? If there is a lot of gold, perhaps there have been many challenges?

The Japanese use the art of 'Kintsugi' to repair broken pottery. They don't see their treasured broken pottery as the end of the object's life, but rather as a defining moment in its lifespan. It is a poetic metaphor for examining our lives don't you think?

Did you ever notice that when you go through a crisis whether small or large, you can't but help being transformed by the trauma? I grew up in Belfast during 'The Troubles' but I haven't let it define my life. What will repair your spirit?

Remember one thing, your brokenness does not define you. You are more than this and at the end of the race you will be pure gold!

You will have lived a life and faced the challenges head on. The cracks are a testament to your life! There is beauty in this. In your history.

References

(1) Marrinan, G. 'Another Zero' 2018. Book Hub Publishing, Galway

(2) https://www2.deloitte.com/za/en/insights/topics/talent/deloitte-millennial-survey-2020.html

Setbacks in Life & Moving Forward

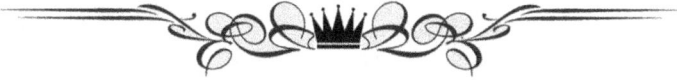

Paul Kilgannon

From the book, 'Be The Best You Can Be In Sport' (Book Hub Publishing, 2020)

'The struggle is the pathway' is a line I often use in my coaching. 'There will be setbacks along the way' is another. Often I quote the former Irish Politician Terence MacSwiney:

"It is not those who can inflict the most, but those who can endure the most who will conquer".

Resilience is the ability to bounce back from adversity and is a crucial quality to develop for sport, and indeed life. Things go wrong in life, in sport. Indeed, much of the story of sport is 'failure', so much so it can be said, that if you are not failing, you are not succeeding. Failing to master a skill instantaneously, reach a goal like a personal best or lose in competition are all part of learning. They are essential for true success, but it must be strongly noted that not all failure leads to success. Progress is never linear. The challenge is always to do what is right even when things are going wrong.

HOW TALENT DEVELOPS

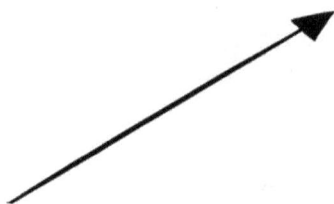

WHAT PEOPLE
THINK IT LOOKS LIKE

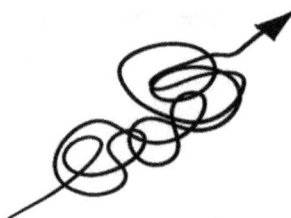

WHAT IT ACTUALLY
LOOKS LIKE.

Adversity can be an important stimulus for growth and development, provided you have the required skills to respond positively and the appropriate support around you. Always seek counsel in times of challenge, talk to trusted adults, coaches, mentors and peers. A problem shared is often a problem halved and the right words, from the right person, at the right time always helps to change focus and strengthen resolve.

Kanter's Law argues that 'Everything looks like a failure in the middle'. 'Expect things to go wrong', may appear negative, or pessimistic, on the face of it, but it is extremely prudent advice. Setbacks are certain but can often be unexpected.

Your focus must always be on how you respond to setbacks and adversity and how you can use it to fuel your subsequent effort and application. Mindset, self-talk and other mental tools and supports we have discussed in the previous chapters, are crucial. Failure is an action and not an identity.

'Failure' can, and should, be productive. In order to grow you must struggle. A prudent way to look at setbacks is that they are happening 'for you, not to you'. The choices we make when we hit obstacles, define us. You can get bitter, or you can get better.

$$E + R = O$$

'Events plus response equals outcome' is another favoured maxim. You must learn to respond to things as opposed to react to them. Fundamentally, you need to be able to treat winning and losing in a similar manner. LOSS- Learning Opportunity Stay Strong. WIN- What's Important Now? Winning and losing is life's ultimate test of character.

When people develop resilience, they condition themselves to respond positively to setbacks and adversity. You can never hide from the fact that in times of adversity, you, and you alone, are in control of how you respond. Welcome your hardships like blessings, for they are laden with opportunity. Adversity can bring opportunity- how you respond to it can be what sets you apart.

In his book Atomic Habits, James Clear writes about a phenomenon of the delay between when we start working toward a goal and the time it takes before we are able to see measurable progress. He refers to this as the 'Plateau of Latent Potential'. It may also be referred to as having the ability to delay gratification. Clear uses the metaphor of the stonecutter pounding away at a rock with seemingly no progress toward his goal, only to finally break the rock with one swing and quotes Jacob August Riis:

"When nothing seems to help, I go and look at a stonecutter hammering away at his rock, perhaps a hundred times without as much as a crack showing in it. Yet at the hundred and first blow it will split in two, and I know it was not that last blow that did it—but all that had gone before".

Breakthrough moments are often the result of many previous actions which viewed incorrectly can be viewed as 'failures'. Just as the child learns to walk, the tripping leads to the walking and builds up the potential required to trigger a major change. Progress in any domain is rarely linear and often takes much longer than you expect. This can result in what Clear refers to as the 'valley of disappointment' where people are discouraged. Don't be discouraged. Plan, plot, learn and drive on in the direction of your goals. Never forget:

> *"Many of life's failures are people who did not realize how close they were to success when they gave up".*

— Thomas Edison

Persistence and strategy can change failure into extraordinary achievement. We cannot control the wind but we can adjust the sail.

Control the mind or it will control you. Often, it will seek to catastrophize things. Understand and appreciate whatever meaning is given to an experience, becomes the experience. What meaning are you attaching to setbacks or failures? This meaning can become self- fulfilling. You are not a robot so you can't expect to be super motivated all the time, and this is why clarity on who you are, and what you value is so important. It will act as your spotlight when times are difficult.

Develop your self-discipline. Self-discipline is the ability to do what is right and necessary when it needs to be done. Self-discipline means setting standards for yourself and living by them. It means being self-reliant- it is your decision, your choice. Move forward in the direction of your goals.

Again, your ability to ask yourself prudent questions is a valuable skill and again we return to the value of journaling. Can you ask yourself questions that will direct your attention to what's working, or what might work better, as opposed to what's not? These are what can be termed 'empowering questions'. 'How can I...', 'What can I ....' questions are powerful to change the focus from the failure or setback, or what didn't work. The right questions change your perspective and perspective is critical in times of challenge. If you can reframe and change the way you look at things, the things you look at will change.

Can you look at failure as feedback and can you learn from it? Appropriate questions give the mind direction and focus, and this is what it needs. They get you thinking constructively. Constructive thinking leads to positive feelings, positive feelings lead to action and this action leads to positive results. Successful people are successful because they have a mindset for success even during failure. Examples of empowering questions to ask in times of struggle or adversity are:

- What can I learn from this?
- How can I use these learnings in the future?
- Where is the opportunity in this?
- Why am I going to be better because of this?
- How can I progress from here?
- How far have I come (this is always important to acknowledge in times of struggle) and what do I now need to do to go further?

Another favoured quote of mine is:

"The first quality of a soldier is constancy in enduring fatigue and hardship. Courage is only the second. Poverty, privation and want are the school of the good soldier".

— Napoleon Bonaparte

When training and competing at a high level a strong commitment, discipline, and daily habits are required and can make the difference between success and failure. The higher you go, the tougher the challenges.

Paul Kilgannon

Many days will follow a routine of sleep, eat, school/ work, eat, train, eat, and repeat. While family, teammates, close friends and coaches may understand the demands being placed on you, others may not. They will often question the reason, and motivation, behind choosing such a disciplined lifestyle. Never forget the line from American architect Russell Warren:

"Obsessed is a word used by the lazy to describe the dedicated".

Some people will consciously, or unconsciously, try to pull you down for being different or committed. Aim to surround yourself with people who energise you. Never forget, unusual results begin with unusual behaviours and actions. If you have just suffered defeat in competition, performed poorly, picked up an injury, or even your self-motivation is simply feeling low, it can be a challenge to entertain and answer the typical "I don't know how you do it", or "is it really worth it?" narratives that people can often offer. It is only you that can answer as to whether it is worth it or not.

"If you want to improve, be content to be thought foolish and stupid".

— Epictetus

As has already been noted, being crystal clear on who you are, why you chose to participate in sport and what you gain from it, are vital in holding your resolve and bringing you through your struggles and challenges. Having this knowledge and understanding can also help you to maintain motivation through what can sometimes appear a relentless season, packed with fixtures and competition. Once again, the practice of journaling is an excellent ally here.

It can be difficult, especially if sport becomes more serious, to keep it in the appropriate context. Throughout your youth, and indeed beyond, sport should be something that enhances your life, brings fun, excitement, challenges, friendships, opportunities, successful days and not so successful days. They are all part of the road to enjoyment, excellence and true success. Sport should leave you feeling better for having done it. Do not let it determine what you are or who you are. Sport is not your only identity. It's important to be yourself and to know yourself. As discussed in many of the previous chapters, having a broad and rounded sense of self-identity is helpful when aspects of your sporting life are not going to plan. It can help you on the road to recovery, whether due to injury, poor form or performance. As a well-rounded person you have the competencies required to help avoid the vicious cycle of low self-esteem which can be difficult to break. Once again, we return to one of the central themes of the book, character is the foundation of the athlete.

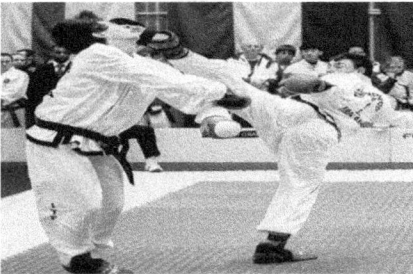

Richie Forde is an ITF Taekwon-Do 5th Degree Black Belt. He was a member of the Irish National Team from 2007 to 2017 and is a World & European Gold Medallist. He is currently Head Coach in East Cork TKD which is home to numerous National and European Medallists. This is his story of overcoming setbacks and failure.

I first made the National Taekwon-Do Team in 2007. Having had much national success, it was time to explore the international circuit. My first taste of the big stage was the 2007 European Championships. I lost in the first round and my championships were over. Later that same year, I travelled to Canada to compete in the World Championships. The result was the same; out in the first round.

The following year came and having gained what I believed to be much experience I felt it was my opportunity to make my mark. The 2008 Euros & World Cup came along and again, I exited in the first round. The story repeated itself in 2009- first round and out!

2010 brought the European Championships in Sweden. Being honest, I didn't really have any great expectations, but I had that dream of being able to stand on that podium hearing Amhrán Na Bhfiann with the Tricolour around my shoulders. That vision was clear in my mind. On this occasion, unlike my previous outings I got my hand raised at the end of the first fight…and the second, and the third.

I had landed myself into a semi-final and I was over the moon as I was guaranteed my first international medal! I came through that semi-final and was now at least guaranteed a silver medal.

After an extremely tough final, it ended in a draw. Extra time also ended in a draw and it went to sudden death. First score wins! The referee signalled to begin and my opponent launched towards me. I instinctively jumped in the air and landed a clean punch on my opponent's face. I fell to my knees with joy! I went from losing in the first round 3 years consecutively to winning my first fight & becoming European Champion in the blink of an eye. So what's to learn from this experience?

Disassociate the Results from your Passion

Looking back on it now I never really lost hope or felt demoralised with losing. Of course, I was disappointed but it never deterred me or stopped me in my tracks. I think there is an important lesson to be taken from this and it is you shouldn't relate your self-worth, or love for something, to results. Do it because you love it, not for any external reasons or recognition from others.

Seek Challenges

Another valuable lesson to take from this is how important experience, learning & challenge are when it comes to reaching your potential in any particular craft. We need to experience hardship of some sort and view them as valuable development opportunities that allow us to challenge ourselves and constantly push forward.

Patience is a Virtue

Those who persevere will be rewarded! Perseverance is one of the guiding principles of Taekwon-Do training. Setbacks are inevitable, it's about how we respond to them. How we perceive setbacks, is what makes the difference. Anything worthwhile should be difficult to achieve! Have a "why" which is strong enough to overcome any setback which may come your way.

I wish you well,
Richie Forde

Chapter Summary Points

- Resilience is the ability to bounce back from adversity and is a crucial quality to develop for sport, and indeed life.
- Failure is a part of learning.
- Progress is never linear.
- Adversity can be an important stimulus for growth and development, provided you have the required skills to respond positively and the appropriate support around you.
- Setbacks are certain but can often be unexpected.

- Fundamentally you need to be able to treat winning and losing in a similar manner. LOSS- Learning Opportunity Stay Strong. WIN- What's Important Now?
- Breakthrough moments are often the result of many previous actions which viewed incorrectly can be viewed as 'failures'.
- Persistence and strategy can change failure into extraordinary achievement.
- The right questions change your perspective and perspective is critical in times of challenge.
- Aim to surround yourself with people who energise you.
- Being crystal clear on who you are, why you chose to participate in sport and what you gain from it, are vital in holding your resolve and bringing you through your struggles and challenges.
- If you can build a 'strong self-image', then mistakes that happen will wash through your mind very quickly. How you talk to yourself during mistakes or after defeats will either add or take from your strong self.

References

(1) Clear, J. (2018). Atomic Habits. UK: Random House.

Releasing Attachment and Welcoming Change

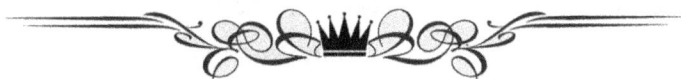

Siobhán Dunleavy

From the book, 'Accepting And Connecting With Muscular Dystrophy'
(Book Hub Publishing, 2021)

I n the months that followed my counselling sessions I was feeling quite content but on the other hand I felt like I was in a bit of a slump. My ego was telling me to settle down, pay my rent, continue to work long hours and do what society was telling me to do but my soul was telling me different. Everyone around me seemed to be settling down and having kids but I wasn't ready for this. I was only in my mid-twenties and even though I was deeply attached to my hometown, the thoughts of settling there at that time, scared the life out of me.

Short holidays and adventures were no longer fulfilling my desires and I craved an adventure as meaningful as the one I experienced in Istanbul. Although I loved and cared deeply for my friends and family it was time for me to spread my wings and continue to follow my own path. I remember reading somewhere at the time "You cannot heal in the same environment that made you sick", and for some reason this touched my heart. I needed to release the attachments I had to my false sense of security in order to move away from the sensations of stagnation that were creeping back into my life. Something was telling me that if I stopped trying to grasp, own and control the world around me I would find more freedom and happiness.

It may sound quite drastic, but I decided to quit my job, give up my house, sell my car and move to Asia. During meditation and in my dreams, I kept having visions of myself being indulged in Asian cultures and gaining more knowledge. I had learned so much but still felt like my soul craved something deeper. The people closest to me probably thought I was mentally mad, but I knew deep down in my soul this is what I was supposed to do. I was also mindful that my muscles were becoming weaker and if I was to travel solo around Asia, I would need to use a walking aid.

As my consciousness grew and my ability to live in the present moment became more natural, using a walking aid no longer felt like such a big deal to me. I knew if I was to follow my true spiritual path there were practicalities that needed to be considered.

It may sound strange but by accepting how Muscular Dystrophy was affecting my life, I became more open to detaching from the body I once had. I wasn't giving up on my body but I was open to finding ways to empower it.

In my late teens and early twenties, I had many falls similar to the ones I described such as the time in Istanbul but as I hit my mid-twenties the falls became more recurrent. It got to a stage where walking on any sort of uneven surface would throw me off my tracks and before I knew it, I'd end up on my arse. These frequent falls were forcing my world to become quite small as more and more I began to avoid situations where I envisioned myself being at risk of falling. What concerned me more than falling and seriously injuring myself was the fear of not being able to get back up onto my feet independently.

There was one fall in particular, that happened not long before I moved to Asia which really helped me to come to my senses. It wasn't pleasant but it was certainly a reality check.

It was a miserable, misty morning in my hometown and I was on the way to get cash out of the ATM on the main street. The disabled parking spot near the machine was being used so I parked across the road. After my not so perfect attempt at parallel parking I grabbed my debit card from the glove box and pulled my hood up to shelter my freshly blow-dried locks from the rain. It was raining that 'wet' type of rain which it does quite often in Ireland. You know where it's not even heavy enough to turn the wipers up full speed but when you're out in it, it subtly sprays onto you and saturates you in seconds. Excuse my French but we often refer to it as 'pissy aul rain'.

I took a deep breath and made my way across the road. The town was fairly quiet and I gathered most people were still at home tucked up in bed dodging the dreary morning. I got about four or five not so sturdy steps across the street when a gust of wind came and threw me off my balance and I crashed to my knees. I hit the ground like a tonne of bricks. The pain that immediately shot up my knees was the least of my worries, I was more concerned about getting a belt of a car. I was slightly relieved when I looked left and right to see there were no cars coming. "Thank fuck for that" I thought to myself as I made an attempt to get back onto my feet.

Although I had been trying to keep my flexibility and my ability to get from the floor to a standing position through yoga and especially the downward facing dog pose, it wasn't happening. I was like a new-born calf who simply hadn't the strength to stand. I had no other choice but to crawl back over to my car. I was fuming as my knees tore off the bumpy concrete on the main street. There must have been no one watching as I imagine they would have helped, although I did look like a bit of a basket case so I couldn't blame anyone for not approaching me. I reached into my pocket for the zapper, unlocked my car, flung the door open and with the support of the seat and the door of my good old Ford Focus I managed to manoeuvre myself onto the driver's seat. The blood was seeping out through my bony knees and new tracksuit bottoms, I clenched onto the steering wheel head butted it almost giving myself a heart attack when I sounded the horn.

What became clear to me from that morning onwards was that my falls had gotten worse and I was no longer sure of being able to get up off the ground independently. This was a serious reality check and sad realisation for me and I knew it was time to invest in a walking aid, even more so if I was to move abroad. I had been winging it for long enough but it had come to a stage where the risk of falling, being seriously injured and being stranded on the ground had to be minimised. It's a scary feeling to be left lying on the ground so helpless and I had to ensure it didn't become a regular occurrence.

After much meditating on things like acceptance, change and self-belief I met with my OT and physio and they provided me with a walker. As much as it was something I wanted to avoid for as long as possible I also knew it wasn't too early to be using it. It's what I needed. I knew that a walking aid would help me to move around with more ease and provide me with a sense of assurance and safety. At this point carrying things whist walking had become especially difficult for me and the walker could make situations like shopping less stressful. I could use the walker to carry my bits and bobs on as well as a support to walk longer distances without falling. When I began using the walker it took me a while to grow fond of it and I would still try to walk short distances without it. For example popping into small shops or appointments where I could get parking near the door.

When I began using my new set of wheels at first, I felt like I was flashing a neon sign to the world that I needed help and my body was different. I certainly found that others began to treat me differently. Moving through doorways, down aisles and through crowds with my walker took a bit of getting used to but I kept reminding myself that we all need help to get through life at some stage or another. Feeling self-conscious about this wasn't an option and I was determined not to let it get in the way of what I needed, especially when I knew it was freedom. I allowed the walker to become a big part of my life but didn't allow it to define me no matter where I went. I don't use my walker at home or in small indoor areas as I can usually move around independently but I've learned to bring it with me, especially in unknown environments. It can always be parked up and left to one side. It's better to have it and not need it than not have it and need it.

It was emotional leaving my loved ones and venturing out to the other side of the world with my relatively new walker but the strength and fulfilment that I got when I landed in Bali, which was the first stop on my big adventure, was liberating. Learning all about Balinese Hinduism reminded me that my soul was doing what it was supposed to and my consciousness and spiritual journey was growing. It took a lot of grounding and mindfulness to stay positive when people would stare at me pushing this walker around, but I would constantly remind myself that I was on my own journey of awakening and nothing was going to stop me. Not the curbs, the inaccessible public transport, the falls, the Bali belly, nor the curious hawk eyes I met every time I ventured outside.

As much as I thought Ireland wasn't accessible Bali and other parts of Asia were ten times worse. The walker was certainly a blessing but it didn't solve all my problems. Walking on uneven surfaces, especially stones, was still very difficult and I needed to avoid them as much as I could. The beach is another place it usually doesn't work well and I tend to stick to the promenades or boardwalks, unless the sand is compacted because then it's not too bad. Time and time again, and even to this day, when I come across paths that have steep curbs instead of slopes to come down off, I often have to risk the danger of walking on the road to get to where I want to be. Although the walker is a fantastic support, it also isn't very useful for walking down steep hills because even though there are breaks on it, it tends to run away from me which can also be lethal.

After my time in Bali, I then went on to travel around Thailand. In Thailand I had the same challenges regarding accessibility and people's reactions, but I welcomed every one of them and was led to endless amounts of opportunities that allowed me to immerse myself into mindfulness and meditation. I stayed in temples and monasteries with Buddhist monks, went on silent meditation retreats, played poker with the mafia of Bangkok, came face to face with my fears, visited temples big and small, took in the beautiful scenery and over all just soaked myself in the magical energy of the country.

After a couple months in Thailand, I then went on to Japan where I would live and work as an English teacher for the following 14 months. When the language school asked me where abouts in Japan I would like to be placed I decided to leave it up to the universe and allow them to choose. It just so happened that the area they sent me to which was called Tokushima, was the starting point for the Shikoku pilgrimage route. This is one of the few circular-shaped pilgrimages in the world. It includes 88 'official' temples and numerous other sacred sites where Ku-kai (Kōbō Daishi) is believed to have trained during the 9th century. He was a renowned monk who established the Shingon (Esoteric) school of Buddhism in Japan during the early Heian era (794-1185). I kid you not, the energy I felt here and the things I learned were not something I could have ever experienced back home.

Once again, by detaching from my comfort zone, my soul had taken me to exactly where I was meant to be. Every day I woke up and looked out over the rice fields I would be absolutely bursting with gratitude and excitement for what the day would bring. Teaching English to Japanese children and adults was an absolute pleasure and I learned as much from them as they did from me. The polite manner and enthusiasm that seeped from my students was invigorating. I often had to pinch myself just to make sure it was real life. As strange as it sounds, teaching English taught me English and the art of linguistics began to fascinate me. My American colleagues, especially Scott, would laugh at how he could barely understand me half the time and he couldn't believe how my students were learning.

I had to retrain my brain to slow down my speech and pronounce my words properly but this didn't stop my students, especially the younger ones picking up the Irish accent. Myself and Scott found ourselves in stitches laughing when the kids would attempt to say things like 'thirty-three' but instead say 'tirty tree'. The pronunciation of my th's never improved, one thing that wasn't capable of changing was my ingrained Irish accent, but I was happy about that.

The sort of spiritual connection I felt in Asia was not something I could easily put my finger on at the time. On reflection I realise that I was almost in my own little world over there but even though I was in my own little bubble I was still making valuable connections. I was able to experience every beautiful moment with a fresh pair of eyes and connect with Asian people as well as other foreigners, this is something I never would have had the chance to do in Ireland. I felt strangely at home there, like there was some sort of weird cosmic relationship between my soul and my surroundings. Obviously not everyone has to live in Asia to move further along their spiritual awakening. This is just a snippet of my journey and nobody else's will be the same. What I hope you can gather though, is that your soul will pull you to places throughout your life and you will probably face lots of challenges along the way, but it's only by taking chances and facing your fears that you can give your soul the opportunity it needs to grow and evolve. It's normal to feel scared and vulnerable when making decisions and setting goals but remember, if your dreams don't scare you, maybe they're not big enough.

Creative Writing

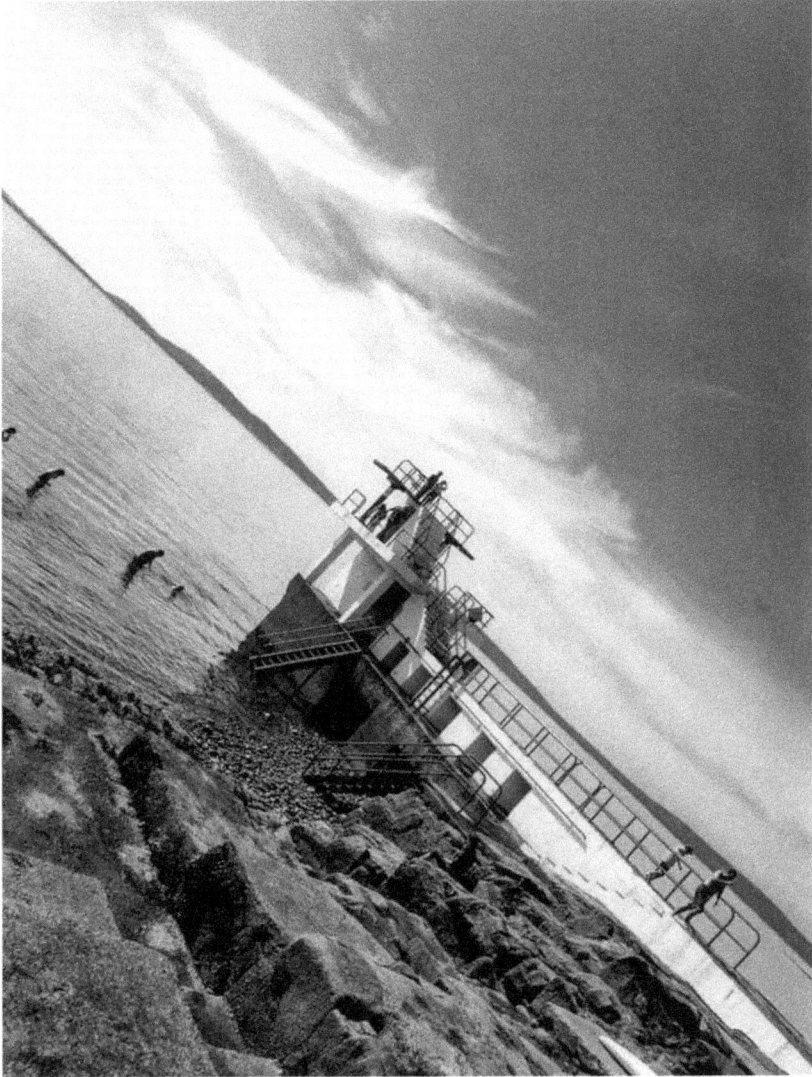

Eighteen

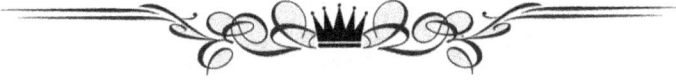

Edel Hanley

At the far end of town I would wait for your arrival at the park gates
a little tired after the working week, but smiling, on Saturdays,
as though I were waiting all day on a platform for the one train
to arrive to carry me away through its cloistered tunnels,
fields of grass, that would stare in from grease-pawed windows,
as an old lady unrolled a newspaper, tutting to herself
as young children passed up and down for the toilet,
clutching hold of bears and Barbie dolls like living things.

And I think again of how much I'd always wanted to leave
this place, growing up, to take off at eighteen and never come back,
believing that all my life something more was somewhere else.
But then I think of you, approaching now, with sleeves rolled up,
eyes watering in the May sun, with daffodil curls blowing away
the ordinariness of these kickabout teenage streets, waving me down
where I decide to tear up my ticket, watching trains pull in and out
like people on the move, the ones forever chasing eighteen.

Moss

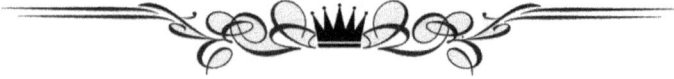

Edel Hanley

There is only a longing, a longing for north and rain,
wherever this inky moss grows, clinging only to the
unsunny walls of the garden, hidden walkways worn
down by our unlooking feet, letting slip a secret
where silence sneaks past, like children's wishes
for adulthood, for something more each time.

Sometimes I wonder how her thick green mattress
survives, finds strength to live in places light fails
and darkness takes over and I want to do the same,
glimpsing my mother bed down snap dragon, curling
delphiniums, her prayer that they do not die blowing
like pollen towards everything, towards the moss.

Perhaps

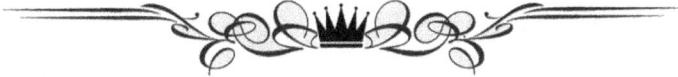

Edel Hanley

Perhaps the waves wind down after all,
lapsing into silence as the morning gulls
fly away, and the fairground closes
its doors for the night.

Perhaps, tonight, you'll sit out and stare
into the void we wanted so desperately
to forget, longing for someone to watch
the curve of night move in

beside you, as summer rain pulsates hard
at your window, like children trying to hide
tears, pressing sticky palms against eyes
fogged with disappointment and regret.

Mental Health

Health

On Wellbeing

FOR
MILLENNIALS
VOL 4

Series Editors
Dr. Niall Mac Giolla Bhuí
And
Dr. Phil Noone

www.ingramcontent.com/pod-product-compliance
Lightning Source LLC
Chambersburg PA
CBHW020457030426
42337CB00011B/138